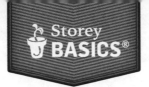

HERBS FOR COMMON AILMENTS

How to Make and Use Herbal Remedies for Home Health Care

Rosemary Gladstar

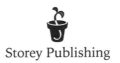

Storey Publishing

*The mission of Storey Publishing is to serve our customers by
publishing practical information that encourages
personal independence in harmony with the environment.*

Edited by Deborah Balmuth and Melinda A. Sheehan
Series design by Alethea Morrison
Art direction by Cynthia N. McFarland and Jeff Stiefel
Text production by Theresa Wiscovitch
Indexed by Nancy D. Wood

Cover illustration © Meg Hunt
Interior illustrations by Alison Kolesar, 37; Beverly Duncan, 15, 19, 29, 45, 50,
51, 64, 68, 71, 95, 99; Charles Joslin, 89; Judy Eliason, 91; Mallory Lake, 55;
and Sarah Brill, 42, 52, 57, 59, 87

Storey books are available at special discounts when purchased in bulk for premiums
and sales promotions as well as for fund-raising or educational use. Special editions or
book excerpts can also be created to specification. For details, please send an email to
special.markets@hbgusa.com.

Storey Publishing
210 MASS MoCA Way
North Adams, MA 01247
storey.com

Storey Publishing, LLC is an imprint of Workman Publishing Co., Inc., a subsidiary of
Hachette Book Group, Inc., 1290 Avenue of the Americas, New York, NY 10104

ISBNs: 978-1-61212-431-5 (paperback); 978-1-61212-432-2 (ebook)

Printed in the United States by Versa Press on paper from responsbile sources
10 9 8 7

LIBRARY OF CONGRESS CATALOGING-IN-PUBLICATION DATA ON FILE

CONTENTS

ACKNOWLEDGMENTS

There is a circle, green hands enfolded, lives entwined, of fellow herbalists. I've held each of their hands and laughed and prayed with them, these old friends who influenced my earliest teachings. Their thoughts are embedded in my heart and flow into the words of this book.

It has been over three decades since we first met at the earliest herb gatherings in Sonoma County. We offered some of our original herb classes and went on some of our earliest herb walks together. At a time when herbalism wasn't popular or faddish, we "followed our bliss," our green passion. Now practically elders, ever more impassioned by the green world, we face a new millennium, wondering not what the world has in store for herbalism but what the herbs have in store for us.

You always run the risk of forgetting someone very important as the night lights fade and the years draw on, but for this moment, I'm remembering these faces from 30 years ago: Svevo Brooks, Nan Koehler, Rob Menzies, Jeannie Rose, Drake Sadler, Ed Smith, Christopher Hobbs, Michael Tierra, Sara Katz, Gabrielle Howearth, James Green, Kathi Keville, Ryan Drum, Mindy Green, Steven Foster, Mark Blumenthal, Warren Raysor, Nam Singh, David Winston, and several who have already crossed "the great divide" — Cascade Anderson Geller, Jesse Longacre, Selena Heron, Jeannine Parvati Baker, Gail Ulrich, and Michael Moore.

May the circle ever grow and the weeds be plentiful.

CHAPTER ONE

UNDERSTANDING HERBS

I was at a large conference a few years ago participating in a panel of "experts" on herbal medicine. Each person on the panel had been involved in herbal studies for more than two decades and was quite well known and knowledgeable about the subject. It was a long workshop, with discussions on different aspects of herbal medicine. I think we all felt fairly good about the perspectives we were sharing and the overviews we had given, but when it came time for questions and answers, the very first question came from a woman sitting in the front row. She stated quite simply, "I came here hoping to gain some clarity about how to use herbs for myself and my family, and now I'm more confused than ever." This book is written for her.

CHOOSING HERBAL MEDICINE

WITH ALL THE POSSIBLE OPTIONS offered by health care today, making a wise choice can be challenging. What is the most responsible thing to do? Each situation is different and warrants a different approach. In one instance antibiotics and a hospital visit may be a wise choice; in another situation herbal remedies and home treatments may be the most responsible approach to take. So how do you decide?

Basically, if your grandmother would have treated the problem at home, you probably can too. This is a sweeping statement, I know, and there are many exceptions to it. Though herbalism can be, and is, effectively used for complex health situations, even life-threatening situations at times, it is best as a home health care system.

Most illnesses and imbalances respond to nourishment, rest, and gentle natural treatments. If your body does not respond in an appropriate manner or does not respond quickly enough for the situation, then consider consulting a medical practitioner, ideally one who is interested in and knowledgeable about holistic treatments. Keep in mind that unless health care practitioners are educated about herbs, they will not be able to give you good advice on the use of herbs, and most practitioners will instruct you not to use them simply because they aren't familiar with most herbs' effects.

When to Use Herbs

Each situation requiring medical attention is different, and each of us as individuals responds differently to treatment. But here are some guidelines for recognizing when herbal treatments can be a better choice than allopathic medical treatments:

As preventive medicine. Herbs are inimitable for building and strengthening the body's natural immunity and defense mechanisms. They nourish the deep inner ecology of our systems on a cellular level. Herbs are also powerful adaptogens, increasing the body's ability to adapt to the ever-changing environment and stressors of life. Having evolved with herbs for thousands of years, our bodies have an innate familiarity with them, recognize them on the deepest levels, and efficiently utilize them.

For most nonemergency medical situations. Everyday problems such as bruises, swellings, sprains, cuts, wounds, colds, fevers, and mild (first degree) burns respond well to herbal healing. Herbs can also be an effective, "on the spot" first aid treatment for emergency situations in which medical help is unavailable or on its way.

As therapeutic agents. If you choose to undergo more radical forms of treatment for serious illnesses such as cancer, AIDS, multiple sclerosis, and other autoimmune disorders, herbs serve as excellent secondary therapeutic agents, supporting and replenishing the body's life energy. Herbs and allopathic medicine work compatibly in these critical situations and can be used to complement and enhance the effects of one another.

Complementing Allopathic Health Care

Herbalism and allopathic medicine often seem at odds with one another. But they are, in fact, complementary and work together quite compatibly. Whereas allopathic drugs actively kill bacteria and viruses, herbal medicines build and restore the system. Allopathic medication generally has a specific agenda; herbs, through a complex biochemical process, take the whole person into consideration and replenish the body at a cellular level. When taken correctly, herbs do not upset the body's innate sense of harmony, so there are few or no side effects. Using herbal therapies to complement pharmaceuticals often helps eliminate or lessen the side effects of drug therapies.

Though some of the strongest herbs should not be used in combination with allopathic drugs, most herbs do not interfere with the actions of pharmaceuticals and can safely be used to augment allopathic treatments. (None of those "strong" herbs are called for in this book.) There is a growing body of information about drug/herb interactions, but it's important to note that most of this research is in its infant stage. People react differently to both herbal medicine and pharmaceutical medicine. Because of this, whenever you're considering using herbal medicine but you're also taking a pharmaceutical, you should consult with a holistic health care professional, who knows and understands herbal medicine, to determine if herbs are recommended in your situation.

Getting Perspective on Herb Safety

Herbs are among the safest medications available on earth. This does not mean that there are not toxic plants or herbal remedies that can cause side effects or harmful reactions in the body. But herbalism as a system of healing has been practiced for several thousand years. The herbs we use today have been used for centuries by people around the world.

Herbs that have toxic side effects have been noted and well documented; wisely, most of these herbs are not available for sale in this country. Occasionally an herb will stimulate an idiosyncratic reaction in an individual. This doesn't make the herb toxic, just a poor choice for that particular individual. Strawberries, a perfectly delicious fruit, are sweet nectar to some and a noxious substance to others. Wheat, another perfectly benign food, is an allergen to a large number of people and can cause dire consequences in a few.

There are many reports surfacing these days about the toxicity of herbs. Even perfectly benign substances such as chamomile and peppermint are finding themselves on the "black list." I think the reason for this is not that more people are using herbs, as is often suggested, but that people are using herbs in ways that allow greater and more concentrated dosages. In the past, herbs were most often taken as teas and syrups, in baths and salves, and in tinctures and extracts. But herbal capsules, which allow people to swallow greater amounts, and standardized preparations, which are far beyond the normal concentrations found in nature, have not been available until recently.

Any herb, even the safest and most researched of herbs, can affect different people differently. Though it is a rare occurrence, a negative reaction to herbs is often reported in the news and soon makes national headlines, creating a certain alarm among plant users. Were drug reactions reported with the same fervor, we'd have a national headline on aspirin every day. However rare these reactions to herbs may be, it is always wise to practice caution when using an herb for the first time, especially when administering to children.

With millennia of experience behind the use of medicinal herbs, their safety is assured. Follow the appropriate dosages outlined in this book (see page 25), use only those herbs that have a record of safety, and respond quickly by discontinuing an herb if you suspect that it is causing a negative response.

The Safety of Medicinal Herbs

Each year approximately 100,000 people in the United States die from adverse reactions to legally prescribed drugs, making them the fourth leading cause of death among Americans. In addition, over 2 million serious but nonfatal problems are caused annually by pharmaceuticals. If there were any deaths due to the use of medicinal herbs, they were not reported. The American Association of Poison Control Centers (AAPCC) receives so few toxicity reports from medicinal herb usage that there is no special category assigned to them. The AAPCC reports that herbs are not a major public health hazard, while houseplants and mushrooms account for a great number of poisonings each year, as do prescription and over-the-counter drugs.

CHAPTER TWO

THE ART OF MAKING HERBAL REMEDIES

It took years to develop the recipes and formulas in this book, and it is with pleasure that I pass them along to you. When I first began working with herbs in the late 1960s, what little explanation there was on how to prepare herbs was difficult to find. Often the steps were complicated, and sometimes the herbs mentioned were not even available. Through a creative process of trial and error, learning from the old masters and their books, and sharing with and learning from friends, the instructions for these preparations began to take shape. Included in this chapter is the information I wish I had when I first began to study herbs.

BUYING AND STORING HERBS

IT IS IMPORTANT TO INSIST ON high-quality, ideally organically grown herbs. Though these herbs may cost a few cents more, they are far better for our medicines and, ultimately, our planet. Have on hand at all times at least 2 ounces of the herbs you plan to use. And don't use herbs either from this country or elsewhere that are endangered or at risk in the wild. It is critical when using herbs today that each person takes responsibility for where the herbs are coming from and who is growing and harvesting them. To learn more about endangered herbs, contact the United Plant Savers (see Resources on page 120).

Purchasing Herbs

How do you tell if a dried herb is of good quality? It should look, taste, and smell almost exactly as it does when fresh, and it should be effective. Dried herbs should have vibrant color, and though they may not necessarily smell "good," they should smell strong. They should also have a distinctive, fresh flavor. Again, they may not taste "good"; judge their taste by potency rather than flavor. If you find one of your herbal remedies is not effective, look to the quality of the herbs you used in making it.

I have traveled widely, and I am astounded by the differences in the quality of herbs in different parts of the world. In the early days of herbalism in the United States, the quality of our herbs was very poor, but over the last three decades, there has been such an emphasis on using high-quality herbs that we now lead the world in quality standards.

We are hoping to have the same influence worldwide on the preservation of medicinal plant populations. If we wish to preserve this system of healing for our children, protecting medicinal plant species becomes imperative. You are supporting not only your own health but the health of the planet when you buy organic and sustainably harvested herbs.

Growing Your Own Medicinal Herbs

The best way to assure you're getting quality herbs is to grow your own. Many of the plants that you use for medicine can be grown as part of your vegetable and flower garden. Incorporate them into your landscape and use them as they grow and thrive. Most herbs are exceptionally easy to grow. For complete instructions, read Tammi Hartung's excellent book *Homegrown Herbs* (Storey Publishing, 2011).

Many of the at-risk medicinal plants have specific habitats and limited range, which is one reason why they are threatened. They can be challenging but extremely rewarding to grow. An excellent guide to growing such at-risk herbs is Richo Cech's book *Growing At-Risk Medicinal Herbs: Cultivation, Conservation, and Ecology* (Horizon Herbs, 2002).

Storing Herbs

Herbs retain their properties best if stored in airtight glass jars, away from direct light, in a cool area. For convenience, you can store them in many other containers — boxes, tins, plastic bags — but most conscientious herbalists find durable glass bottles the best for storage.

Each herb has its own shelf life, and following a set rule could mean you would throw out perfectly fine peppermint while using poor-quality chickweed. As previously described, you can quickly determine whether a particular herb has retained its quality: Does it smell strong? Is its color vivid? Does it taste fresh? If so, despite what the books say about shelf life, it is probably still good. The final test is always effectiveness: does it work?

THE KITCHEN "LAB"

A KITCHEN, WITH ALL OF ITS marvelous tools, will supply you with most of the utensils you need for preparing herbal products. One of the few rules that most herbalists agree on is never to use aluminum pots and pans for preparing herbs. Despite its popularity, aluminum is a proven toxic substance that is easily released by heat. Instead, use glass, stainless steel, ceramic, cast iron, or enamel cooking equipment.

Here are some items I've found especially useful:

- Cheesecloth or fine muslin for straining herbs
- A large, double-meshed stainless steel strainer
- Stainless steel pots with tight-fitting lids
- A grater reserved for grating beeswax
- Canning jars of various sizes for storing herbs and making tinctures
- Measuring cups (though, heaven forbid, I hardly use them)
- A coffee grinder for grinding herbs (Don't use your herb grinder for coffee; you'll forever have the flavor of herbs in your coffee and the scent of coffee in your herbs.)

HOW TO DETERMINE MEASUREMENTS

WHILE MANY PEOPLE ARE converting to the metric system, I've reverted to the simpler's method of measuring. Many herbalists choose to use this system because it is extremely simple and very versatile. Throughout this book you'll see measurements referred to as "parts": 3 parts chamomile, 2 parts oats, 1 part lemon balm. The use of the word "part" allows the measurement of any one ingredient to be determined in relation to the measurement of the other ingredients. The "part" can be interpreted to mean a cup, an ounce, a pound, a tablespoon, or what-have-you — as long as you use that unit consistently throughout the recipe. If you were using tablespoons in the recipe above, you would measure out 3 tablespoons of chamomile, 2 tablespoons of oats, and 1 tablespoon of lemon balm. If you were using ounces as your unit of measurement, you'd use 3 ounces of chamomile, 2 ounces of oats, and 1 ounce of lemon balm. See how easy it is?

HERBAL TEAS

HERBAL TEAS REMAIN MY favorite way of using herbs medicinally. The mere act of making tea and drinking it involves you in the healing process and, I suspect, awakens an innate sense of healing in you. Though medicinal teas are generally not as potent or as active as tinctures and other concentrated herbal remedies, they are the most effective medicines for chronic, long-term imbalances. And all you really need to make them is a quart jar with a tight-fitting lid, your selected herbs, and water.

Herbal teas can be drunk hot, at room temperature, or iced. They can be made into ice cubes with fresh fruit and flowers and used to flavor festive holiday punches. They're delicious blended with fruit juice and frozen as pops for children.

Once brewed, an herbal tea can sit at room temperature for quite some time, but after several hours or when left out overnight, it will eventually go "flat," get tiny bubbles in it, and begin to sour. Stored in the refrigerator, an herbal tea will keep for 3 to 4 days.

I seldom direct people to make medicinal teas by the cupful. It is impractical and time consuming. Instead, make a quart of tea each morning or in the evening. Use 4 to 6 tablespoons of herb per quart of water. The herb-to-water ratio varies depending on the quality of herbs, on whether the herbs are fresh or dried (use twice as much fresh herb in a recipe), and on how strong you wish the tea to be. There are two basic methods for making tea, and two variations I've included just for fun.

Infusions

Infusions are made from the more delicate parts of the plant, including the leaves and flowers. Place the herb in a quart jar (or any container with a tight-fitting lid), and pour boiling water over the herb. Cover, and let steep (infuse) for 30 to 45 minutes. A longer steeping time will make a stronger tea. Strain, reheat if needed, and your tea is ready to drink. For medicinal purposes it is always recommended to drink your herbal tea (or any liquid, for that matter) warm or at room temperature.

Decoctions

Decoctions are made from the more tenacious parts of the plant, such as the roots and bark. It's a little harder to extract the constituents from these parts, so a slow simmer (or an overnight infusion) is often required. Place the herb in a small saucepan and cover with cold water. Heat slowly, and simmer with the lid on for 20 to 45 minutes. Again, the longer you simmer the herbs, the stronger the tea will be. Strain and drink.

Solar and Lunar Infusions

Have you ever considered using the light of the moon or the sun to extract the healing properties of herbs? It's one of my favorite methods for making herbal tea. Sometimes, after I've prepared a tea on my kitchen stove, I'll place it in the moonlight or sunlight to pick up some of the rays of these giant luminaries. We are children of the sky as well as the earth; using the energies of the stars, moon, and sun in our healing work adds a special touch.

Solar tea is made by placing the herbs and water in a glass jar with a tight-fitting lid. Place directly in the hot sunlight for several hours.

Lunar tea is made by placing the herbs and water in an open container (unless there are lots of night-flying bugs around!) and positioning it directly in the path of the moonlight. Lunar tea is subtle and magical; it is whispered that fairies love to drink it.

SYRUPS

Syrups are the yummiest of all herbal preparations, and children often prefer their medicine in this form. They are delicious, concentrated extracts of the herbs cooked into a sweet medicine with the addition of honey and/or fruit juice. Vegetable glycerin may be substituted for honey; it is an excellent medium for the herbs and is very nutritious.

HOW TO MAKE SYRUP

This is my favorite method for making syrup.

Step 1. Combine the herbs with water in a saucepan, using 2 ounces of herbs per quart of water. Over low heat, simmer the liquid down to 1 pint. This will give you a very concentrated, thick tea.

Step 2. Strain the herbs from the liquid. Compost the herbs and pour the liquid back into the pot.

Step 3. Add 1 cup of honey (or other sweetener such as maple syrup, vegetable glycerin, or brown sugar) to each pint of liquid.

Step 4. Warm the honey and liquid together only enough to mix well. Most recipes instruct you to cook the syrup for

20 to 30 minutes longer over high heat to thicken it. It does certainly make thicker syrup, but I'd rather not cook the living enzymes out of the honey.

Step 5. When the syrup is finished heating, you may add a fruit concentrate to flavor it; or perhaps a couple of drops of essential oil, such as peppermint or spearmint; or a small amount of brandy to help preserve the syrup and to aid as a relaxant in cough formulas.

Step 6. Remove from the heat and bottle for use. Syrups will last for several weeks, even months, if refrigerated.

Though you can make almost any herb or herbal formula into a syrup, the most popular syrup, without question, is elderberry syrup. You can make elderberry syrup using either fresh or dried berries. (For more on elder, see page 38.)

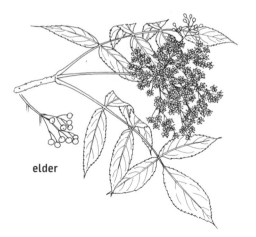

elder

HERBAL CANDY

FAR MORE DELIGHTFUL THAN taking herbs in tinctures or pill form are these delicious medicinal candies. You can mix just about any herbal formula this way.

HOW TO MAKE HERBAL CANDY

Step 1. Grind raisins, dates, apricots, and walnuts (the exact proportions are up to you) in a food processor. Alternatively, you can mix nut butter (such as peanut, almond, or cashew) with honey in equal portions. (If you're concerned about the use of honey, then use maple syrup, rice syrup, or maple cream.)

Step 2. Stir in shredded coconut and carob powder, again in whatever proportions you like.

Step 3. Add your herbs, in powdered form. Mix well.

Step 4. Roll the mixture into balls. (To yield the recommended dosage, divide the amount of herbs you've used by the dosage, and roll that number of balls. For example, if you've used 10 teaspoons of herbs, and the dosage is ½ teaspoon, you'd roll 20 balls.)

Step 5. Roll the balls in powdered carob or shredded coconut. Store in the refrigerator.

HERBAL PILLS

HERBAL PILLS ARE simple, practical, and easy to make. You can formulate your own blends and make them taste good enough so that even children will eat them. Formulate them with herbs for the throat to make a tasty sore throat remedy to suck on.

HOW TO MAKE HERBAL PILLS

Step 1. Place powdered herbs in a bowl and moisten with enough water and honey (or pure maple syrup) to make a sticky paste.

Step 2. Add a tiny drop of essential oil, such as peppermint or wintergreen oil, and mix well.

Step 3. Thicken with carob powder, adding enough to form a smooth paste. Knead until the mixture is smooth, like the texture of bread dough.

Step 4. Roll into small balls the size of pills. You can roll them in carob powder for a finished look if you like. (To give each the recommended dosage, divide the amount of herbs you've used by the dosage, and roll that number of pills. For example, if you've used 10 teaspoons of herbs, and the dosage is ½ teaspoon, you'd roll 20 pills.)

(continued on next page)

Step 5. Place the pills on a baking tray and set to dry in the oven at very low heat (even the pilot light will work), or just in the sun. These pills, once dried, will store indefinitely. I often store mine, undried and unrolled, in the refrigerator, in a glass jar with a tight-fitting lid, and roll them as I need them.

MEDICINAL OILS

HERBAL OILS ARE SIMPLE to make and may be used on their own or as a base for salves and ointments. By using different combinations of herbs and oils, you can make either strong medicinal oils or sweet-scented massage and bath oils. Though any good-quality vegetable oil may be used, the oil of choice for medicine is olive; there is simply no finer oil for this purpose.

If your herbal oil grows mold, there is either too much water content in the herb or too much moisture in the jar. Use dried herbs or wilt the herbs before using. Be *absolutely* certain the container is completely dry. Check the lid for moisture; it is often the culprit.

Making Solar-Infused Oils

Place the herbs and oil in a glass jar; cover tightly. Place the jar in a warm, sunny spot. Let the mixture infuse for 2 weeks, after which you may strain the oil, add a fresh batch of herbs, infuse for 2 more weeks, and strain again. This will give you a very potent medicinal oil. Use cheesecloth or a muslin cloth to strain the oil, squeezing out the spent herbs to extract every last drop of oil.

Using the Double-Boiler Method

Although it doesn't provide the benefits of the sun, this is a quick and simple method that makes beautiful oil.

Place the herbs and oil in a double boiler and bring the water in the lower pot to a low simmer. Gently heat the oil for 30 to 60 minutes, checking frequently to be sure it is not overheating. The lower the heat and the longer the infusion, the better the oil.

Next, strain the oil. Line a large stainless steel strainer with cheesecloth or muslin and place it over a large bowl. Pour the mixture through. Reserve the oil.

Storing Herbal Oils

Store your finished herbal oil in a cool, dark area. It does not have to be refrigerated, but it will quickly deteriorate in heat. Stored properly, herbal oils will last for several months, sometimes even years.

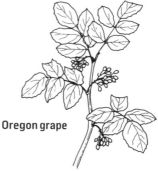

Oregon grape

SALVES AND OINTMENTS

ONCE YOU'VE MADE HERBAL oil, you're a step away from a salve. Salves and ointments (basically different terms for the same product) are made of beeswax, herbs, and vegetable (or animal) oils. The oil is used as a solvent for the medicinal properties of the herbs and provides a healing, emollient base. The beeswax also adds a soothing, protective quality and provides the firmness necessary to form the salve.

HOW TO MAKE A SALVE

Step 1. Prepare a medicinal oil, following the instructions on pages 18–19.

Step 2. To each cup of herbal oil, add ¼ cup beeswax. Heat until the beeswax is completely melted. To check the firmness, place 1 tablespoon of the mixture in the freezer for just a minute or two. If it's too soft, add more beeswax; if it's too hard, add more oil.

Step 3. Pour the mixture into small glass jars or tins. Keep one out for use, of course, and store any extra in a cool, dark place. Stored properly, salves will last for months, even years. Some people recommend adding natural preservatives to the mixture, such as vitamin E or tincture of benzoin, but I've never found it necessary or any more effective.

TINCTURES

TINCTURES ARE CONCENTRATED extracts of herbs. Most tinctures are made with alcohol as the primary solvent or extractant. Alcohol is a strong solvent and extracts most of the important chemical constituents in plants. Effective tinctures can also be made with vegetable glycerin or apple cider vinegar as the solvent. They are not as strong as alcohol-based preparations, but they do work, and some people who choose not to use alcohol-based tinctures may prefer them. Because of their sweet nature, glycerin-based tinctures taste far better than those made with alcohol, and they have a longer shelf life.

Some of the alcohol in tinctures can be removed by placing the tincture in boiling water for 1 to 2 minutes. This method is only effective for removing about 50 percent of the alcohol; some residual alcohol will always remain.

Herbal Liniments?

An herbal liniment is made in exactly the same way as a tincture; however, a liniment, which uses rubbing alcohol or witch hazel as its solvent, is for external purposes. Liniments are used either for disinfectant purposes or to soothe sore, inflamed muscles.

To make a liniment, follow the directions on pages 22–23, simply substituting for the solvent. Be sure to label the bottle FOR EXTERNAL USE ONLY *to avoid accidents.*

Several methods can be used to make tinctures. The traditional or simpler's method is the one I prefer. It is an extremely simple system that produces beautiful tinctures every time. All that is required to make a tincture in the traditional method is the herbs, the solvent, and a jar with a tight-fitting lid.

HOW TO MAKE A TINCTURE

Step 1. Chop your herbs finely. I recommend using fresh herbs whenever possible. High-quality dried herbs will work well also, but one of the advantages of tincturing is the ability to preserve the fresh attributes of the plant. Place the herbs in a clean, dry jar.

Step 2. Pour the solvent over the herbs. If you're using alcohol, select one that is 80 to 100 proof, such as vodka, gin, or brandy. If you're using vegetable glycerin, dilute it with an equal amount of water before pouring it over the herbs. If you're using vinegar, warm it first to facilitate the release of herbal constituents.

Completely cover the herbs with the solvent and then add an additional 2 to 3 inches of liquid. The herbs need to be completely submersed. Cover the jar with a tight-fitting lid.

Step 3. Set the jar in a warm place and let the herbs and liquid soak (macerate) for 4 to 6 weeks — the longer, the better. Place the jar where it will demand daily attention, such as on a kitchen windowsill, or even in the bathroom.

Top off the jar with additional solvent as needed, to maintain that 2 to 3 inches of coverage over the herbs. I encourage shaking the jar of tincture daily during the maceration period. Shaking your tincture not only prevents the herbs from packing down on the bottom of the jar but is also an invitation for some of the old magic to come back into medicine making. While shaking it, you can sing to your tincture, stir it in the moonlight or the sunlight, wave feathers over it — whatever your imagination inspires.

Step 4. Strain the herbs from the solvent by pouring the mixture through a large stainless steel strainer lined with cheesecloth or muslin. Reserve the liquid, which is now a potent tincture, and compost the herbs. Rebottle and be sure to label it, or you'll quickly forget what's in the jar. Include the name of the herb, the solvent used, and the date. Store in a cool, dark location, where the tincture will keep for a year or more.

To take a dose of tincture, simply dilute a dropperful or two in warm water or juice and drink it.

HERBAL BATHS

THERE ARE SEVERAL PROMINENT healers who administered most of their herbal formulas via the bath. Depending on the herbs or herbal formulas you choose and the temperature of the water, you can create either a relaxing bath or a stimulating, uplifting one, or a bath that is soothing, or decongesting, or good for depression. Herbal baths open up the pores of the skin, our largest organ of elimination and assimilation. Bathing is nothing less than immersing yourself in a strong infusion of healing herbal tea.

The water should be warm or hot for a relaxing bath, cool to cold for a stimulating bath, and tepid for a neutral bath. Place the herbs in a large handkerchief, clean nylon stocking, or strainer, and tie it on the nozzle of the tub. (There are also large stainless steel strainers made exactly for this purpose; look for them in your local herb or kitchen shops.) Allow the hot water to flow through the herb bag until the tub is half filled. Adjust the water temperature as desired and fill the tub the rest of the way.

Herbal baths may also be administered solely to the feet or hands. All of the nerve endings in the entire body pass through the feet and hands, making them a map of our inner being.

Dosage Guidelines

Chronic problems are long-term imbalances such as PMS, chronic back pain, migraines, arthritis, and allergies. They usually develop slowly over a period of weeks or months and generally require a long-term commitment to correct the imbalance. Chronic problems can flare up and manifest acute symptoms, but the underlying problem is long-standing.

Acute problems come on suddenly, reach a crisis quickly, and need immediate response. Acute problems can be toothaches, headaches, menstrual cramps, and burns. Pain is often an acute symptom, but it can be caused by either an acute or a chronic problem.

PREPARATION	DOSAGE FOR CHRONIC CONDITIONS	DOSAGE FOR ACUTE CONDITIONS
Tea	3–4 cups daily for 5 days, rest for 2 days, then repeat for several weeks, or until the problem is corrected	¼–½ cup throughout the day, up to 3–4 cups, until symptoms subside
Extracts or tinctures*	½–1 teaspoon 3 times daily for 5 days, rest for 2 days, then continue for several weeks, or until the problem is corrected	¼–½ teaspoon every 30–60 minutes until symptoms subside
Capsules or tablets	2 capsules/tablets 3 times daily for 5 days, rest for 2 days, then continue for several weeks, or until the problem is corrected	1 capsule/tablet every hour until symptoms subside

*Includes syrups and elixirs.

Note: Though it's not necessary to follow an exact cycle of 5 days on and 2 days off, I've found that herbs work better when you don't use them every day; this pattern mimics the natural cycle of renewal. Some herbalists follow a cycle of 3 weeks on and 1 week off.

CHAPTER THREE

THE HOME HERBAL PANTRY

Though it's always a challenging task to decide which of the many wonderful herbs to include in listings such as this, I've limited my discussion to those herbs that have the greatest safety record and are commonly used for household situations. Most of these herbs can be used successfully over a long period of time, with no harmful side effects, and for a variety of purposes. Warnings are given where appropriate. For a more complete listing of beneficial herbs or for further information on the herbs that I have included, consult any one of the encyclopedic herbal compendiums available today.

Reading will fill your head with the wonderful facts and stories about each plant, but herbalism is more than "head" learning. Plants teach by interacting with us, so the best possible way to learn about each herb is to experience it. When teaching my students how to use herbs, I insist they try each one as a tea. In this way, they learn about its flavor and effects. Next, I ask them to research the herb in at least three good reference books to get a variety of thoughts and opinions about each plant. This information augments their direct experience with the herbs.

After you've read about it, if it seems like an appropriate herb for your situation, try it. The taste, the smell, the effect of the herb on your being is the best laboratory you have for determining its effectiveness. Listen to the wisdom of your body, the feeling of the herb as you're using it, and the book knowledge you gain as you read about it.

Astragalus (*Astragalus membranaceous*)

PARTS USED: roots

BENEFITS: Adaptogenic, tonifying, and sometimes referred to as "the young person's ginseng," astragalus strengthens the deep immune system and helps rebuild the bone marrow reserve that regenerates the body's protective shield. It is particularly beneficial for strengthening the spleen and lungs. It is a superior tonic herb and is used in the treatment of chronic imbalances. It is also useful for regulating the metabolism of dietary sugars, and thus it is helpful for people with diabetes.

SUGGESTED USES: Astragalus is best used in tea for long-term illness, for low energy, and to support and build deep immune strength. Astragalus can also be used in capsule form. Or just eat it as is: place a whole root or two in a pot of soup and simmer for several hours, or chew on it like a licorice stick; it's quite tasty.

Burdock (*Arctium lappa*)

PARTS USED: primarily the roots and seeds, but the leaves can be used externally

BENEFITS: This tenacious wild plant is a bane to farmers and a blessing to herbalists. It is simply the best herb for the skin and can be used internally and externally for eczema, psoriasis, acne, and other skin-related imbalances. It is a superior tonic herb for the liver, and because of its pleasant flavor it is often formulated with other less tasty "liver herbs."

SUGGESTED USES: Burdock makes a fine-tasting tea; teenagers with problem skin could try it mixed with juice or other herbal teas. It is also used as a wash for itchy, irritated skin. Decoct the root and serve with meals as a digestive aid. The fresh root, grated and steamed and served with a sprinkle of toasted sesame seed oil, is delicious. The seeds are often used in ointments for the skin.

Calendula (*Calendula officinalis*)

PARTS USED: flowers

BENEFITS: Known to most people as marigold or pot marigold, this sunny little flower brightens most gardens. It is a powerful vulnerary (heals wounds), healing the body by promoting cell repair, and acts as an antiseptic, keeping infection at bay. Calendula is often used externally for bruises, burns, sores, and skin ulcers. It is also used internally for fevers and for gastrointestinal problems such as ulcers, cramps, indigestion, and diarrhea. It is also a wonderful lymph tonic and is cleansing and strengthening for the immune system. And, of course, you see it used in many cosmetics for its skin-soothing and beautifying effects.

SUGGESTED USES: Calendula is most often used in salves for burns and irritated skin, but it is also effective as an infusion for skin problems, fevers, and gastrointestinal upsets. It is oftentimes brewed as a triple-strength tea and used as a hair rinse. For use as a lymph tonic, try a calendula tincture (see How to Make a Tincture, pages 22–23).

calendula

Cayenne pepper (*Capsicum annuum* and related species)

PARTS USED: fruits

BENEFITS: Cayenne is beloved around the world, with almost a cultlike following. And it's really quite deserving of all the attention it gets. Not only a wonderful fired-up culinary herb used in all manner of dishes worldwide, it is also a highly valued medicinal plant. It serves as a catalyst to the system, stimulating the body's natural defense system. It has antiseptic properties and is an excellent warming circulatory herb. It is one of the best heart tonics, increasing the pulse and toning the heart muscle. Cayenne is also a natural coagulant that stops bleeding. Finally, it is an excellent carminative, stimulating the digestive process and helping with congestion and constipation.

SUGGESTED USES: Cayenne can be used sparingly in many formulas (teas, capsules, tinctures, and food preparations) as a catalyst or action herb. The burning feeling it creates is superficial and not harmful.

CAUTION: Cayenne, though perfectly safe, is hot. Even a pinch of cayenne in a tincture formula can overwhelm, and a grain or more in an herbal pill can send you to the ceiling! Use with caution and only in small amounts. Always wash your hands well with soap and water (or vegetable oil or cream) after working with cayenne so as not to transfer it to your eyes.

Chamomile (*Anthemis nobilis* and related species)

PARTS USED: primarily the flowers, but the leaves are useful

BENEFITS: This little plant is a healing wonder. In its flower tops, it has rich amounts of a deep blue essential oil called azulene that acts as a powerful anti-inflammatory agent, making chamomile excellent for relieving pain in joint problems such as arthritis and bursitis. Its flowers make a soothing tea that is relaxing for the nervous systems. It is a general digestive aid and is one of the best herbs for colicky babies.

SUGGESTED USES: The tea sweetened with honey can be served throughout the day to calm stress and nervousness. A few drops of chamomile tincture will aid digestion and is excellent for calming babies. Chamomile makes a wonderful massage oil for relieving stress and anxiety; the herb and its essential oil are often used in oils and salves for sore, achy joints. Chamomile is also found in many cosmetic formulas, as it aids in skin repair, and it is also frequently added to bathwater for a wonderfully relaxing and soothing wash.

Chaste tree (*Vitex agnus-castus*)

PARTS USED: berries

BENEFITS: Chaste tree, a shrub native to the Mediterranean region, has been employed by Europeans since ancient times. It is one of the most important herbs for feeding and nourishing the reproductive organs of both men and women and is especially helpful in restoring vitality and general tone to the female system. Chaste tree is the herb of choice for many women to relieve the symptoms of menopause and PMS and to regulate any kind of menstrual dysfunction. (While chaste tree is an important herb for many women, it doesn't work for everyone; pay attention when first using it to see if it's the right choice for you.) Many people use it to enhance their sexual vitality, though there's some controversy about whether it stimulates or depresses sexual desire. I find it to be amphoteric in action, meaning that it stimulates or depresses depending on what your body needs, while addressing the root cause of the imbalance.

SUGGESTED USES: Chaste tree berries look and taste a bit like black pepper. Though they can be camouflaged in tea, they are most often used in tincture or capsule form. They can also be put in a pepper grinder and used like pepper.

Chickweed (*Stellaria media*)

PARTS USED: aerial parts

BENEFITS: Chickweed can be found worldwide in moist, cultivated soil and is commonly considered a weed. It is highly esteemed for its emollient and demulcent properties and is a major herb for skin irritations, eye inflammation, and kidney disorders. It is often used in salves and poultices for rashes and other skin irritations. It is a mild diuretic and is indicated for water retention. In addition, chickweed is a treasure trove of nutrients, including calcium, potassium, and iron.

SUGGESTED USES: The fresh tender greens are delicious in salads. They can also be juiced; they're particularly good blended with pineapple juice. A light infusion of chickweed is wonderfully soothing. This herb doesn't dry or store well, so to preserve it for future use, try tincturing some of the next crop of chickweed that pops up in your garden. Rather than view it as a weed, see it as the healing, tender, and tenacious little plant it is.

Cleavers (*Galium aparine*)

PARTS USED: aerial parts

BENEFITS: Another common garden weed, cleavers is often found growing near chickweed; they seem to enjoy the same habitat. And the two are often combined in formulas as well. Both cleavers and chickweed are mild, safe diuretics, and both are used to tone and soothe irritations of the kidneys and urinary tract. In addition, cleavers is an excellent lymphatic cleanser and is often used as a safe, effective remedy for swollen glands, tonsillitis, and some tumors.

SUGGESTED USES: Prepare in the same way as chickweed. Cleavers also does not dry or store well, so prepare it as a tincture for future use.

Coltsfoot (*Tussilago farfara*)

PARTS USED: leaves

BENEFITS: Its botanical name, *Tussilago*, means "cough dispeller," and coltsfoot has long been cherished as a remedy for coughs, colds, and bronchial congestion. It is an antiasthmatic and expectorant, helping to dilate the bronchioles and expel mucus. Coltsfoot is a common weed found growing along roadsides, ditches, and streams throughout the United States. People often confuse it with dandelion, as the flowers are similar. But coltsfoot blooms in the very earliest part of spring, before the large, rounded leaves appear.

SUGGESTED USES: Coltsfoot is often infused with other compatible lung herbs, such as mullein, sage, elecampane, and wild cherry, and served as a tea.

CAUTION: There is some concern about the safety of *Tussilago* because some members of the large family to which it belongs have been found to contain PLAs, a group of chemicals that can cause damage to the liver. Studies have been inadequate and inconclusive, and none show coltsfoot to be harmful or damaging. Because of these findings and because coltsfoot has been used safely and effectively for hundreds of years, I continue to use it.

Comfrey (*Symphytum officinale*)

PARTS USED: leaves, roots

BENEFITS: Rich in allantoin and deeply healing, comfrey is commonly used in soothing poultices, salves, and ointments. It facilitates and activates the healing of tissue. It is absolutely one of the best herbs for torn ligaments, strains, bruises, and any injury to the bones or joints. It can also be used internally; rich in mucilage, it soothes inflammation in the tissues when administered as a tea or in pills.

SUGGESTED USES: The root and the leaf have similar properties; the root is stronger, the leaf is more palatable. Use them both in salves and ointments. The root is decocted, the leaf infused.

CAUTION: As with coltsfoot, studies several years ago found traces of PLAs in comfrey. The studies weren't conclusive, and I, personally, along with many other herbalists, continue to use comfrey, though I don't use it in formulas meant for internal use by others. You can decide for yourself whether you feel comfortable ingesting comfrey. However, comfrey is absolutely safe to use for external purposes; everyone agrees on this!

Corn silk (*Zea mays*)

PARTS USED: golden (not brown) silk of corn

BENEFITS: The corn silk (flower pistils) from maize has long been used as a urinary tonic. It acts as an antiseptic, diuretic, and demulcent on the urinary system. It will stimulate and clean urinary passages while soothing inflammation. It is one of the most effective herbs for counteracting bed-wetting and incontinence. Corn silk is also, surprisingly, delicious, tasting a bit like fresh corn on the cob.

SUGGESTED USES: Use as a tea during the day to strengthen the urinary system. Take corn silk as a tincture at night to help prevent bed-wetting. Other treatments, such as Kegel exercises, should be used in conjunction with corn silk for the treatment to be most effective.

Dandelion (*Taraxacum officinale*)

PARTS USED: entire plant

BENEFITS: Half the world loves this plant, using it for medicine and dining on it daily. The other half has been trying to destroy it with chemical warfare since the 1940s. But dandelion's tenacity is part of its beauty and, perhaps, has something to do with its medicinal properties. The roots are a superior liver tonic and can help relieve poor digestion and lower bowel complaints. The leaves are a mild diuretic used to treat water retention and bladder or kidney problems. They are rich in iron, calcium, and other trace minerals and are treasured the world over as delicious wild greens. The flowers make a delicious wine.

SUGGESTED USES: Dandelion root is decocted and served as a tonic tea for the liver. The root, when tender, can be chopped like a carrot and added to a stir-fry or soup. The leaves are infused for tea, steamed, or added raw to salads. Dandelion has a bitter zest to it, so it's best when blended with milder herbs. My favorite way to eat the leaves is to steam them and then marinate them overnight in Italian dressing and honey.

Echinacea (*Echinacea angustifolia, E. purpurea,* and related species)

PARTS USED: roots, leaves, flowers

BENEFITS: This beautiful, hearty plant is among the best immune-enhancing herbs that we know of and one of the most important herbs of our time. Though incredibly effective, it is not known to have any side effects or residual buildup in the body. Echinacea works by increasing macrophage T-cell activity, thereby increasing the body's first line of defense against colds, flus, and many other illnesses. It is also an excellent herb for the lymphatics. Though potent and strong, it is 100-percent safe, even for young children and the elderly.

SUGGESTED USES: Take echinacea in frequent small doses in tea or tincture form to boost immunity at the first sign of a cold or flu. It is also useful for bronchial infections as a tea or tincture. Use as a spray for sore throats. For sore gums and mouth inflammation, make a mouthwash from the root, with peppermint or spearmint essential oil to flavor it.

CAUTION: Several species of echinacea are used for medicinal purposes, and even more species are common ornamental

Echinacea Mouthwash

To make a refreshing and healing herbal mouthwash, prepare echinacea root as a tincture (follow the instructions on pages 22–23). Combine 4 ounces of the tincture with 3 ounces of water and a couple of drops of essential oil of peppermint or spearmint. Mix well. To use: Add 1 to 2 teaspoons of the tincture to half a glass of warm water. Swirl it around in your mouth several times and spit it out. Repeat as needed.

varieties in the garden. *Echinacea purpurea* and *E. angustifolia* are the two most commonly used medicinal species. Because of its popularity in both Europe and the United States, echinacea has been poached extensively from the wild and is now considered an at-risk herb by the United Plant Savers (see page 120). Thankfully, many organic farmers are now growing it. Help us save our native species by using echinacea only from organically cultivated sources, and avoid using wild-harvested echinacea.

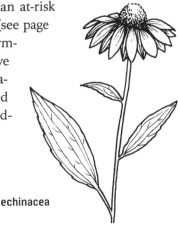

echinacea

Elder (*Sambucus nigra*)

PARTS USED: berries, flowers

BENEFITS: Elder flower syrup is Europe's most esteemed formula for colds, flus, and upper respiratory infections. You can find this tasty product in most pharmacies as well as natural food stores throughout Europe. In the United States, elderberry syrup and tincture are also popular remedies for flu and cold viruses, though you are more apt to find them in herb and natural food stores than in pharmacies. Both the flowers and berries are powerful diaphoretics: by inducing sweating, they reduce fevers. Elder has powerful immune-enhancing and antiviral properties as well and is even more effective when combined with echinacea.

SUGGESTED USES: Elderberries make some of the best syrups and wines you'll ever taste. The flowers are also edible and medicinal and are often used in teas for fever. Every summer I collect the large, fragrant flat clusters of elder flowers and make elder flower fritters as a special summer treat. Served with elderberry jam, elder flower fritters are especially divine.

CAUTION: There are a few different varieties of elder that grow in the United States. Those with blue berries are safe to eat, though most people agree that it's best not to eat the fruit raw but to cook, dry, or tincture it. The berries of red elder, a small shrub that grows in higher elevations and looks similar to the blue elder, except for its bright red fruit, are not edible. Don't eat red elderberries!

Elecampane (*Inula helenium*)

PARTS USED: roots

BENEFITS: A large sunflower-like plant, elecampane is easily grown in any garden, but watch out! It can take over. Elecampane's large root has long been used for deep-seated bronchial infections. It serves as an excellent expectorant (helps expel mucus from the lungs) and a stimulating respiratory tonic, and it is one of the most popular herbs for coughs, bronchitis, asthma, and chronic lung ailments. Though a powerful and effective medicinal plant, it is safe to use.

SUGGESTED USES: Elecampane is frequently combined with echinacea to combat bronchial infections, and because of its soothing properties it is frequently combined with licorice to treat irritation and inflammation in the lungs. Elecampane can be made into a tincture using either the fresh or the dried root. It is also effective as a tea (decoction) or capsule.

Fennel (*Foeniculum vulgare*)

PARTS USED: primarily the seeds, but the leaves and flowers are tasty and useful as well

BENEFITS: A popular carminative and digestive aid, fennel was used by the early Greek physicians for all manner of digestive problems and also to increase and enrich milk flow in nursing mothers. It is an effective antacid, both neutralizing excess acid in the stomach and reducing uric acid from the joints, thus helping to fight inflammation. Fennel seeds are a popular remedy for digestion, and relieve flatulence. They also help regulate and moderate appetite. They can also be used to relieve colic.

SUGGESTED USES: With their licorice-like flavor, fennel seeds are quite tasty and are often combined with other less flavorful herbs to make formulas more palatable. They can be prepared as a tea to relieve colic, improve digestion, and expel gas from the system. (Remember, however, that the gas doesn't disappear but is *expelled*, so you may be tooting a bit!) Nursing moms can drink 2 to 3 cups of fennel tea daily to increase the flow of their milk. Fennel tea also makes a soothing wash for soreness and inflammation in the eyes, and it can be combined with infection-fighting herbs like goldenseal to treat conjunctivitis and other eye infections. (Remember, however, to strain the fennel tea well so as not to get any herb particles in your eyes.)

Feverfew (*Tanacetum parthenium*)

PARTS USED: leaves, flowers

BENEFITS: This common garden flower has an outstanding reputation for the treatment of migraines. Recent pharmacological studies have proved that it also alleviates inflammation and stress-related tension.

SUGGESTED USES: Because it is quite bitter, I generally combine feverfew with lavender and California poppy to make a tincture. As a migraine preventive, take ½ to 1 teaspoon of the tincture two to three times daily for 5 days, rest for 2 days, and then repeat the cycle. Feverfew is most effective for managing migraines when taken over a period of 2 to 3 months, though it will also alleviate acute migraine symptoms if taken at the very earliest signs of a migraine. While it is best to tincture the herb fresh, I've found that high-quality, properly dried feverfew works as well.

Garlic (*Allium sativum*)

PARTS USED: bulbs

BENEFITS: Garlic! What *isn't* there good to say about garlic? One of the oldest and most popular kitchen/herbal remedies, garlic may be one of nature's great gifts to humankind. Rich in sulfur compounds and volatile oils, garlic is a potent infection-fighting herb and can be used both externally and internally. It has both antiviral and antibacterial properties, which makes it a great remedy for fighting off colds and flus. It is also rich in immune-enhancing properties, which stimulate the immune system to ward off invading pathogens. Garlic is a well-known vermifuge and has a long history of being used to prevent and treat worms and parasites in animals as well as people. Garlic is also renowned for its ability to promote healthy cholesterol levels and to lower high blood pressure. In addition to all of this, garlic is just plain tasty.

SUGGESTED USES: Contrary to popular opinion, cooking garlic destroys little of its medicinal properties. According to the latest studies, the active ingredients may diminish a bit with cooking, but are still present. Add garlic to your meals. It can be eaten raw by blending it into pesto and dips. I tincture garlic, pickle it (with tamari and vinegar), and make herbal oils with it. It's one of the main ingredients in fire cider, a well-known herb vinegar formula that's packed full of warming, spicy herbs.

Ginger (*Zingiber officinalis*)

PARTS USED: roots

BENEFITS: Recognized as both an important culinary and a valuable medicinal plant, ginger is, like garlic, another of the common, versatile, and extremely useful kitchen remedies. Ginger is a primary herb for the reproductive, respiratory, and digestive systems. It is one of the main ingredients in reproductive tonics for men and women and helps improve circulation to the pelvis. It is a safe and effective herb for motion sickness and morning sickness. It is also a favorite home remedy for menstrual and muscle cramps and tension. A warming and stimulating diaphoretic, ginger opens up the pores and promotes sweating, in this way helping the body to "sweat out" a fever. It is also commonly served as a warming digestive aid before and after meals.

SUGGESTED USES: Ginger is rich in volatile oils and, although it's a root, is best infused. Grated ginger makes a delicious tea with lemon and honey. Ginger powder can be added to many formulas or used in cooking. Try making ginger syrup; it is simply delicious. Hot poultices of ginger can be applied over the pelvic region to help with cramps and stomach tension.

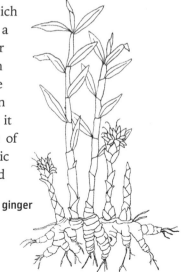

ginger

Ginkgo (*Ginkgo biloba*)

PARTS USED: leaves, fruit

BENEFITS: One of my favorite trees, ginkgo is a slow-growing large perennial tree that can live to a hardy old age. It is the sole survivor of the oldest known tree genus, *Ginkgoaceae*, which dates back over 200 million years. And perhaps its status as a veritable living fossil accounts for its remarkable ability to help with memory and recall. Ginkgo serves as a "brain food" and is a great memory aid. It also enhances vitality and improves circulation. I suggest gingko as a regular tonic herb for anyone experiencing memory loss or "brain fatigue." In recent studies, it has been shown to halt the progression of Alzheimer's when administered in therapeutic dosages (i.e., standardized extracts) over a period of time. Ginkgo must be used with consistency for several weeks before you will notice its benefits.

SUGGESTED USES: Use the standardized capsules or extracts when treating memory loss or early-onset Alzheimer's disease. To strengthen the mind and circulation, in general, ginkgo is effective as a tea, a tincture, or capsules.

CAUTION: Because of its effects on the blood and circulatory system, ginkgo should be discontinued for 2 weeks before and after surgery. Though it's not generally a problem in such cases, it's better to err on the side of caution.

Goldenseal (*Hydrastis canadensis*)

PARTS USED: roots, leaves

BENEFITS: This is quite possibly one of the most useful and valuable plants of North America. Particularly effective at healing mucous membranes, goldenseal is used in cleansing washes for the eye, as a douche for infections (careful: it can be too drying for the vagina if not formulated correctly), in mouthwashes for sore mouths and gums, and in the topical treatment of eczema and psoriasis. It has antibiotic, antibacterial, and antiseptic properties and is often combined with other infection-fighting herbs to help combat infections and ward off colds and flus. Note: Goldenseal is on the United Plant Saver's At-Risk List (see page 120); use only organically cultivated varieties of this endangered plant.

SUGGESTED USES: Goldenseal is very bitter and is often used as a bitter tonic and digestive aid. The root is infused (not decocted) as a bitter tea, which can be used as a mouthwash for gum infections and as a topical wash for cuts. The root is often powdered and used in poultices for infections, abscesses, and wounds. Combine the herb with echinacea to help fight off infections and colds.

CAUTION: If used over a period of time, goldenseal becomes an irritant to the mucous membranes, causing inflammation and irritation. Always rotate its use (for instance, 5 days on, 2 days off), and do not use for longer than 3 weeks at a time.

Hawthorn (*Crataegus* species)

PARTS USED: fruits, flowers, leaves

BENEFITS: Hawthorn is quite possibly the best heart tonic herb there is. It has been revered and surrounded by legend for centuries and is used as a healing plant in every country it grows in. Hawthorn dilates the arteries and veins, allowing blood to flow more freely by releasing cardiovascular constrictions and blockages. It lowers blood pressure while strengthening the heart muscle. It also helps maintain healthy cholesterol levels. Hawthorn is outstanding at preventing heart problems and treating heart disease, edema, angina, and heart arrhythmia. Because it is considered a food rather than a medicine, it is generally considered safe to use in combination with heart medication. But if you're taking any kind of pharmaceutical, you should of course check with your health care professional before using herbs.

SUGGESTED USES: Hawthorn is delicious as a tea, syrup, and jam, and it can also be tinctured. I use powdered hawthorn as a sprinkle on cereal and in blender shakes. It will have best effect if used on a regular basis.

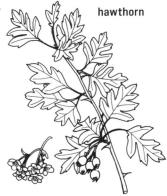

hawthorn

Hibiscus (*Hibiscus sabdariffa* and related species)

PARTS USED: flowers

BENEFITS: Hibiscus is high in vitamin C, bioflavonoids, antioxidants, and a host of other vitamins and minerals. With its rich, bright red pigment, it advertises its own affinity for the heart, and, indeed, it is a good heart tonic. It also has slightly astringent properties.

SUGGESTED USES: The large tropical flowers make a bright red tea that is tasty and tart, with a sweet aftertaste. Hibiscus is often formulated with stevia or other sweet herbs to enhance its flavor. It brightens any tea with its beautiful ruby red coloring. Children especially love hibiscus. Try making a thick hibiscus syrup and add it to sparkling water for a delicious punch. Loaded with vitamins and minerals, this beverage is far better than sugar-loaded soda.

Lavender (*Lavandula* species)

PARTS USED: flowers

BENEFITS: Native to the Mediterranean, lavender blesses us with its beauty and fragrance. While most people think of lavender as only a pretty garden plant, it is actually quite valuable as a medicinal and has been used for centuries for its calming, nervine properties. Beautiful, fragrant, and hardy, lavender is a strong nervine and a mild antidepressant, and it is a wonderful aid for headaches. Combined with feverfew, it helps alleviate migraines. It is one of the most popular herbs to add to the bath for relieving tension, stress, and insomnia. The essential oil is excellent for insect bites, bee stings, and burns (mix with honey). Aside from smelling lovely, the essential oil is also a powerful disinfectant and is a favorite scent in cleansers and soap.

SUGGESTED USES: Add small amounts to tea (its flavor can be overpowering). It makes a tasty glycerin- or alcohol-based tincture. The essential oil is popular in baths and can be used as aromatherapy to soothe the nerves. For headaches, apply two to three drops of the essential oil to the temples and nape of the neck. Apply the essential oil topically for insect bites, prepare as a wash for cuts, or use in the bath, in salves, or as a steam to relieve congestion.

Lemon balm (*Melissa officinalis*)

PARTS USED: leaves

BENEFITS: Calming, antiviral, and antiseptic, this beautifully fragrant and tasty member of the mint family is one of nature's best nervine herbs. When applied topically, lemon balm can help heal and prevent herpes. It is often made into a cream for this purpose, though I find the tincture works as well. Lemon balm tea is used as a mild sedative to ease insomnia and mild depression. It is renowned for lifting the spirits and driving away melancholy.

SUGGESTED USES: Lemon balm makes a delicious tea that can be served with lemon and honey to alleviate stress and anxiety. For a delicious nervine tonic, blend equal amounts of lemon balm, oats, and chamomile. Lemon balm makes one of the tastiest tinctures, in either alcohol or glycerin.

Licorice (*Glycyrrhiza glabra*)

PARTS USED: roots

BENEFITS: The effective and delicious qualities of licorice help make it one of our most important herbal remedies. It is used for a multitude of situations, including bronchial congestion, sore throat, and coughs, and serves as a powerful antiviral medicine for herpes, shingles, and other viral infections. With its amazing mucilaginous properties, licorice can help heal inflammation of the respiratory system and digestive tract and is soothing and healing to ulcers. It is excellent for toning the endocrine system and is a specific herbal remedy for adrenal exhaustion. Because of its soothing and strengthening properties, licorice is a favorite herb of singers. In traditional Chinese medicine, licorice is considered a "superior medicine" and is used as a harmonizer in many formulas.

SUGGESTED USES: Licorice is quite sweet and must be blended with other herbs to be palatable. Though most people enjoy the flavor and taste of licorice, some people have a strong aversion to it. Licorice is often made into syrups and teas. As a tea, it can be made into a wash or poultice for viral infections such as herpes and shingles. For adrenal exhaustion, tiredness, and fatigue, drink 2 to 3 cups of licorice tea a day, blended with other endocrine tonic herbs such as wild yam, sarsaparilla, burdock root, and sassafras. For sore throats, prepare licorice as a cough syrup; combine it with pleurisy root and elecampane for deep-seated bronchial inflammation, and combine it with marsh mallow root for digestive inflammation and ulcers. Licorice can be used in tinctures and capsules, but because of its sweet flavor and soothing mucilaginous consistency, it really shines in teas and syrups.

CAUTION: While generally considered safe — safe enough even for children — licorice is not recommended for individuals who have high blood pressure and/or suffer from water retention. People who are taking heart medication should check with their health care professional before using licorice root.

Marsh mallow (*Althaea officinalis*)

PARTS USED: primarily the roots, but the leaves and flowers are useful

BENEFITS: Marsh mallow belongs to the large Malvaceae family, which also includes hibiscus and hollyhock. It is a particularly benevolent family; it has no toxic members, and many of the "malvas," are used for food and medicine. Marsh mallow is one of the more famous members of this family. The Romans considered its root to be a tasty vegetable, and the sweet leaves were considered a culinary treat among many ancient cultures. Early pioneers in the United States boiled the powdered root with sugar to make a sweet confection, which later morphed into the marshmallow we know today. (Sadly, the modern confection is completely devoid of the herb for which it is named.) A soothing, mucilaginous herb, marsh mallow makes a tasty tea for sore throats, respiratory inflammation, and digestive issues. It is excellent for helping to soothe and heal ulcers and other inflammatory conditions. It is also particularly beneficial for treating urinary tract infections and urinary issues, and in these cases it is frequently combined with other urinary tonics such as chickweed and cleavers.

SUGGESTED USES: Serve as a tea or syrup for sore throats, diarrhea, constipation, urinary tract infections, and bronchial inflammation. The powdered root and/or leaf can be mixed into a paste with water for soothing skin irritations. Marsh mallow along with oatmeal can also be used in the bath for a soothing wash. Marsh mallow can be tinctured, but its mucilaginous constituents are more soluble in water than in alcohol, so water preparations such as tea and syrup are preferable.

Milk thistle (*Silybum marianum*)

PARTS USED: seeds, leaves

BENEFITS: The seeds of this large wild thistle are nature's best aid for damaged liver tissue. This herb is even used in allopathic medicine (especially in Europe) and is the only agent known to prevent fatal amanita (death cap mushroom) poisoning. It directly stimulates liver function and rebuilds damaged liver tissues. Its tonifying actions make it a valuable component of cleansing programs, and an important supplement for those whose livers have been compromised by illness, hepatitis, or alcoholism. Milk thistle seed is also helpful for the gallbladder and the kidneys.

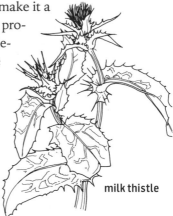

milk thistle

SUGGESTED USES: The hard black seeds should be ground so that the chemical constituents can be more easily drawn out. Use the ground seeds in tinctures or tea, or sprinkle them directly on food. They can be lightly toasted to bring out their rich flavor.

Motherwort (*Leonurus cardiaca*)

PARTS USED: leaves

BENEFITS: Motherwort is best known for its beneficial properties for women, especially for menopausal women, but it's equally beneficial as a heart tonic. Its botanical name, *Leonurus*, means "lionhearted." It is a superb tonic for nourishing and strengthening the heart muscle and its blood vessels. It is a remedy for most types of heart disease, neuralgia, and a rapid heartbeat. It is valued as a remedy for many women's problems, such as delayed menstruation, uterine cramps associated with scanty menses, water retention, and hot flashes and mood swings during menopause. Motherwort grows easily in the garden. It is weedlike and will take over, so be careful!

SUGGESTED USES: Prepare as an infusion flavored with tastier herbs, and drink several cups a day. Or prepare as a tincture.

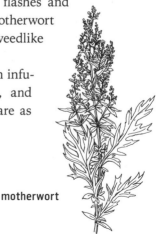

motherwort

Mullein (*Verbascum thapsus*)

PARTS USED: leaves, flowers, roots

BENEFITS: This is one of my favorite wayside weeds. It is always so stately, sometimes sending its flowering stalk several feet high into the sky. That stalk is full of beautiful, fragrant yellow flowers that make the best oil for ear infections. The flowers both fight the infection and relieve the pain. The elongated fuzzy leaves that form a rosette at the base of the plant have been used for centuries in cough formulas and are used for all manner of respiratory and bronchial infections and asthma. The leaves are also excellent for treating glandular imbalances and are indicated whenever there's glandular swelling.

SUGGESTED USES: Mullein leaves and flower can be used in tea, capsule, and tincture form. For bronchial congestion, colds, and coughs, blend the leaves with coltsfoot leaves and peppermint and prepare as a tea. For glandular swelling and endocrine imbalances, mix the leaves with echinacea and cleavers to make an infusion (tea) or tincture. To fight ear infections, prepare a solar-infused oil from the flowers, using olive oil (see page 97 for a recipe).

mullein

Nettle (*Urtica dioica*)

PARTS USED: fresh leaves, young tops

BENEFITS: Often viewed as a pesky plant by gardeners, nettle is nonetheless beloved by herbalists worldwide. It is a delicious wild green when steamed and is a rich source of vitamins and minerals, especially iron and calcium. It is an age-old remedy for allergies, hay fever, and respiratory infections. Because of its nutrient density, and especially its biochelated calcium, nettle is excellent for children and is especially recommended for growing pains, when their bones and joints ache. An excellent reproductive tonic for men and women, nettle is used for alleviating the symptoms of PMS and menopause, as well as for improving fertility in both men and women when the infertility is due to poor nutrition. Nettle is also famous as a hair and scalp tonic; it is said to preserve a full head of healthy hair.

SUGGESTED USES: Nettle is a pleasant-tasting green and is often served steamed. It can be used to replace spinach in any recipe but must always be well steamed; if undercooked, it will sting you! It is also delicious as a tea, which can be served several times a day to prevent allergy attacks. Freeze-dried nettle capsules have the best reputation for treating allergies and hay fever, but I often combine the capsules with tea. Nettle is also effective as a tincture.

Oats (*Avena sativa*)

PARTS USED: green milky tops (but the stems are also useful)

BENEFITS: One of the best nutritive tonics for the nervous system, oats are recommended for nervous exhaustion, stress, and irritation. The plant's mucilaginous properties make it particularly helpful in treating damage to the myelin sheath surrounding nerve fibers. Oats are rich in silica and calcium.

SUGGESTED USES: Oats are best used partially green, before the plant has turned golden. Both the milky green tops and the stalks make a delicious tea — one of the best, I think. Make it strong and mix with fruit juice. The tea works well for people who are nervous, hyperactive, or stressed. You can also use oats to make a wonderfully soothing bath for skin irritations.

Oregon grape (*Mahonia aquifolium*)

PARTS USED: roots

BENEFITS: The roots of this beautiful hollylike plant are gaining fame because they contain berberine, a chemical similar to the active constituent in goldenseal. Oregon grape root is being used in place of goldenseal to help prevent overharvesting of that herb, but Oregon grape is also a slow-growing perennial with a limited growing range. Like goldenseal, Oregon grape root is used both internally and externally to fight infections. It has exceptional anti-inflammatory, antiseptic, and antiviral properties. It is often used in formulas to support liver well being and digestive issues. It's also an important herb for skin problems such as acne, eczema, and psoriasis.

SUGGESTED USES: A decoction of the root can be used as a topical wash for infections. Take it internally for infections, for poor digestion, and as a tonic for the liver.

CAUTION: Whether harvesting it yourself or purchasing it from retailers, be careful to support sustainable practices that limit the risk of overharvesting Oregon grape root. Though often prolific where it is found growing, Oregon grape has a limited range. If wild populations seem to be diminishing, we may determine that this herb be used from only cultivated sources, leaving the wild stands to grow.

Passionflower (*Passiflora incarnata*)

PARTS USED: leaves, flowers

BENEFITS: Passionflower is a beautiful flowering plant known more for its garden appeal than for its medicinal properties. But it is a powerful nervine that has a long history of use for calming and toning the nervous system. Passionflower is an excellent remedy for stress, anxiety, and depression. An effective, gentle

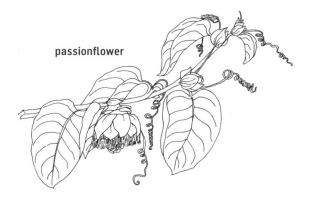

passionflower

herb, it is often recommended for hyperactive children, teenagers, and adults. For many people it's been a helpful remedy for insomnia and other sleep issues.

SUGGESTED USES: The leaves are brewed as an infusion for tea drunk throughout the day. Use the tincture at bedtime to aid in peaceful sleep. The flowers also contain medicinal virtue, but it's difficult to drink something so gorgeous!

Peppermint (*Mentha x piperita*)

PARTS USED: leaves, flowers

BENEFITS: Peppermint has been called a "blast of pure green energy." It's not that there aren't stronger stimulants, but none make you feel so renewed and refreshed. Commonly used as a digestive aid, peppermint is effective for treating nausea, easing stomach cramps, and clearing the mouth of foul tastes. Because of its bright fresh flavor, it's a common ingredient in toothpastes and tooth powders.

SUGGESTED USES: Eat the herb fresh, or prepare as an infusion for sluggish digestion. Use peppermint tea or tincture diluted in water as a refreshing mouthwash. Because of its pleasant, refreshing flavor, peppermint is often used in formulas to help cover up the flavor of less tasty herbs. Though peppermint dries well, it is delicious when freshly harvested from the garden.

Plantain (*Plantago major, P. lanceolata*)

PARTS USED: Seeds, roots, leaves

BENEFITS: Plantain is a common weed found growing throughout the temperate regions of the world. It is often the first plant introduced to children — put it on any "boo-boo" or bee sting and it heals quickly. Plantain is among the best herbs for poultices of all kinds. It's an important herb for treating blood toxicity and blood poisoning and is generally used both internally and externally for this purpose. Plantain seeds are rich in mucilage and are often used in laxative blends for their soothing bulk action. In fact, the psyllium seeds used in Metamucil are produced from a *Plantago* species. This herb is also very effective for treating liver sluggishness and for easing inflammation of the digestive tract.

SUGGESTED USES: Though it is often described as bitter tasting, plantain is quite mild in flavor and makes a nice infusion. It is an excellent herb for poultices for all kinds of skin problems. It can also be powdered and added to food, or used as an herbal first aid powder for infections.

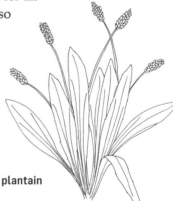

plantain

Red clover (*Trifolium pratense*)

PARTS USED: flowering tops, leaves

BENEFITS: A member of the pea family, red clover has long, thin roots that penetrate several layers of soil and draw up vitamins, minerals, and other elements that are often not found near the surface of the earth. It is renowned for its ability to fix nitrogen in the soil, thereby serving as a natural fertilizer. As a medicinal herb, red clover is one of the best respiratory tonics, useful for young children as well as adults, and it is also one of the best detoxification herbs. It is used for chronic chest complaints such as coughs, colds, and bronchitis. It is used as a tea and as a wash for all skin conditions, and it is commonly found in cancer-prevention and anti-tumor formulas. It is one of the ingredients in traditional anti-cancer formulas such as the Hoxsey formula and Essiac tea.

SUGGESTED USES: Red clover makes a delicious tea. Blend with other herbs such as mullein for persistent respiratory problem, or with nettle as a tea for building the blood and improving the skin. The tea or tincture can be used to prevent and eliminate unwanted growths such as cysts, tumors, and fibroids.

CAUTION: Hemophiliacs, or people with "thin" blood (those who bleed heavily and/or whose blood doesn't clot readily), should not use red clover. It is known as a blood thinner and can promote prolonged bleeding.

Red raspberry (*Rubus idaeus*)

PARTS USED: young shoots, fruits, and leaves

BENEFITS: Raspberry was first cited in Chinese herbal writings dating back to 550 CE. It was also a valuable remedy for the native peoples of the North American continent, who considered it a nourishing tonic and healing remedy for pregnant and nursing women. It has been used as a uterine tonic and nutritive supplement ever since. Raspberry leaves are rich in vitamins and minerals, particularly calcium and iron.

SUGGESTED USES: The leaves, fruit, and young shoots are all used, but the leaf is most often brewed as a tea. Because of its astringent properties, raspberry leaf is valuable for helping to treat diarrhea and dysentery. It helps reduce excessive menstruation and is one of the superior tonics for pregnancy and childbirth. It also makes a good mouthwash for sore or infected gums. It can also be prepared in tincture and capsule form and can be made into a tasty syrup.

red raspberry

Rose hips (*Rosa canina* and related species)

PARTS USED: primarily the seeds, but the leaves and flowers are also useful

BENEFITS: Rose hips contain more vitamin C than almost any other herb, and many times that of citrus fruit, when measured gram by gram. Vitamin C is a noted antioxidant with disease-fighting capabilities. Rose leaves can also be used and are astringent and toning. The lovely fragrant flowers are used in love and heart potions and in many flower essence formulas.

SUGGESTED USES: Make fresh rose hips into a vitamin-rich syrup or jam. Rose hips make a delicious, mild-flavored tea, perfect on a cold night, sipped by a roaring fire. Powdered rose hips can be sprinkled on cereal or in blender shakes. Or try infusing the leaves, hips, and flowers together for a total rose tea.

....

Rose Hip Jam

Rose hip jam is delicious and simple to make. It's best to use dried rose hips, but be sure they are seedless. You can buy dried seedless rose hips, but if you're using your own, either deseed them by hand or press them through a jelly sieve to remove the seeds. Cover the rose hips with 2 to 3 inches of fresh apple juice or cider. Let soak overnight at room temperature. The next morning, you should find that all the juice is absorbed, leaving a thick, sweet, juicy jam in the jar. You can add freshly grated ginger, powdered cinnamon, and other spices, but it's really good enough to eat as it is. Store in the refrigerator.

....

Rosemary (*Rosmarinus officinalis*)

PARTS USED: leaves

BENEFITS: Rosemary is another of our common garden plants that has long been revered for its healing virtues. A renowned memory aid and brain tonic, rosemary has a tonifying effect on the nervous system and is both calming and stimulating. It is an excellent herb for circulation, strengthens the heart, and aids in reducing high blood pressure. It has also been used for hundreds of years as a cosmetic herb for its healthy effects on the hair, scalp, and skin.

SUGGESTED USES: Rosemary is an essential ingredient in the famous gypsy formula known as the Queen of Hungary's Water, a bracing astringent cosmetic preparation. It is effective as a tea, a tincture, or as capsules. It makes a pleasant tea when infused with other herbs and is often blended with ginkgo and gota kola as a memory tonic. Rosemary is also a beloved kitchen herb and is found in a variety of culinary recipes. Use abundantly, not sparingly.

Sage (*Salvia officinalis*)

PARTS USED: leaves

BENEFITS: Sage is another of those kitchen herbs that has a long history of use as a medicinal plant. It's name, *Salvia*, means "to save," perhaps referring to its ability to restore a person to good health. It is an excellent herb for rebuilding vitality and strength during long-term illness. It clears congestion and soothes sore throats, tonsillitis, and laryngitis. It is, in fact, one of the best herbs to use for throat and lung issues, as it is drying, disinfectant, and healing. Sage is frequently recommended for women in menopause to help decrease hot flashes and night sweats.

SUGGESTED USES: Make into a gargle for sore throat and infections in the mouth by soaking sage leaves in vinegar and then adding a little honey and a pinch of cayenne or salt. An infusion of sage is pleasant, warming, and pungent. Perhaps because of its grounding nature, sage is helpful for menopausal women, most specifically for hot flashes. And, of course, sage is excellent as a culinary herb and enhances the flavor of many foods.

St. John's wort (*Hypericum perforatum* and related species)

PARTS USED: leaves, flowers

BENEFITS: Although it has been used for centuries for nerve damage and is held in high esteem by herbalists, St. John's wort was just recently "rediscovered" for its antidepressant activities. It is effective against mild depression and seems to lift the spirits when used on a regular basis. It is a wonderfully safe and effective herb for nerve damage, stress, anxiety, depression, and personality disorders. The beautiful red oil made magically from the cheerful yellow flowers is a wonderful aid for trauma and is one of the best topical remedies for bruises, sprains, burns, and injuries of all kinds.

SUGGESTED USES: Definitely make St. John's Wort Oil; it is one of the finest medicinal oils. The flowers and leaves can also be tinctured or prepared as an infusion (use approximately 70 percent flowers to 30 percent leaves).

CAUTION: St. John's wort causes photosensitivity (sensitivity to the sun) in some individuals. Then again, many people use the oil as a sunscreen to protect themselves from sunburn. I would recommend that anyone taking standardized St. John's wort, which is often a highly potenized form of the herb, avoid exposure to direct sunlight.

There was some earlier concern that St. John's wort worked as an MAO inhibitor, similarly to Prozac, but there isn't sufficient evidence to support this. The action of St. John's wort is not completely understood, but recent studies show that it is not an MAO inhibitor, and, therefore, the restrictions imposed on Prozac users do not apply to those taking St. John's wort.

......

St. John's Wort Oil

St. John's Wort Oil is best made from fresh plant material. Collect the fresh flowers just as the buds are opening, in early to midsummer. If they're ready, they should stain the tips of your fingers bright red when you squeeze them. Collect a few leaves as well; I generally suggest making the oil with roughly 70 percent flowers and 30 percent leaves.

Allow the buds and leaves to air-dry in a warm, shaded area for a few hours. Though this isn't always necessary, it allows some of the moisture to evaporate, and most importantly, it's a polite way to give whatever tiny creatures have made their home in the flowers an opportunity to escape.

Place the buds and leaves in a glass jar, cover with 2 to 3 inches of olive oil, seal the jar, and allow to infuse in a warm, sunny spot for 2 to 6 weeks. The oil should be blood red. Strain, rebottle, and use as needed.

......

Saw palmetto (*Serenoa repens*)

PARTS USED: berries

BENEFITS: This is the herb supreme for men, and for women as well, though it is especially popular among men over 50. Doctors may even recommend it to their male patients as a tonic and preventive herb for prostate health, as well as a specific remedy for enlarged prostate glands. Not so well known are its benefits for women. It firms sagging breast tissue and is an excellent herb for those who are thin and unable to gain weight.

SUGGESTED USES: The berries are pungent and strong tasting, with an oily coating; nothing seems to mask their rather unpleasant flavor. Because of that flavor, saw palmetto is used primarily in tinctures and capsules and not very often in tea.

Siberian ginseng (*Eleutherococcus senticosus*)

PARTS USED: roots

BENEFITS: More than a thousand scientific studies confirm this herb's remarkable properties for enhancing physical and mental performance. Also known as eleuthero, Siberian ginseng has adaptogenic and tonic properties similar to those of *Panax* ginseng. Siberian ginseng strengthens the nervous, endocrine, and immune systems and restores energy and

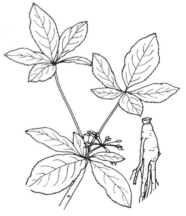

Siberian ginseng

vitality. This is one of the "longevity herbs" made famous in Asia for its seeming ability to promote and sustain a vital long life.

SUGGESTED USES: Use as a long-term tonic. The powdered herbs can be taken in capsule form or added to tonic recipes, blender drinks, and cereal. The root is decocted as a tea. The root can also be dried, chopped, and added to soup (remove the chunks before eating, as they stay hard).

Spearmint (*Mentha spicata*)

PARTS USED: leaves, flowers

BENEFITS: Cooling, refreshing, and uplifting, spearmint is one of the most popular of all the mints. It has a cool, refreshing flavor, milder than that of peppermint. Sometimes called the "mother of all mints," spearmint is often combined with other herbs to make them more palatable. It is a common ingredient in mouthwashes, toothpastes, and breath mints.

SUGGESTED USES: Use to "sweeten" the stomach and breath after sickness, especially vomiting; just add a drop of the essential oil to water or make a cup of fresh tea, and use the liquid to rinse out your mouth. Add spearmint to herb blends, honey, or culinary dishes for a quick, flavorful pick-me-up.

Stevia (*Stevia rebaudiana*)

PARTS USED: leaves

BENEFITS: Called "sweetherb," stevia is 50 times sweeter than sugar but is much better for you. It has no calories and doesn't promote tooth decay. It is indicated for pancreatic imbalances and high blood sugar levels, and it is a type of sugar that diabetics can readily tolerate. In fact, stevia is used to help treat diabetes. Imagine a sweetener that is good for diabetics! Though stevia has been tested extensively in other countries, it was banned in the United States on the pretext that its safety was unknown. But once the sugar industry became involved and secured an interest in stevia production, stevia quickly became legalized, and stevia products began appearing on market shelves.

SUGGESTED USES: Because of its intense sweetness, stevia is primarily used to enhance the flavor of herb teas. But beware, only a small amount will do! If you add even a pinch too much to a cup of tea or to a recipe, you'll ruin the flavor. To control the sweetness, I suggest making stevia no more than 2 percent of the total formula.

Usnea (*Usnea barbata*)

PARTS USED: lichens

BENEFITS: It is odd that an herb so abundant and so useful was not used by modern American herbalists until just a few years ago. Usnea is the lichen that grows primarily on aging trees and is often called "old man's beard"; since several lichens are called by this name, be sure the one you are using is usnea. Containing the bitter usnic acid, usnea soothes the stomach while enhancing digestion. It has antibiotic properties, making it useful for treating urinary and bladder infections, cystitis, and fungal infections. It is an excellent immune enhancer and is frequently combined with echinacea.

SUGGESTED USES: I often add a small amount of usnea to soup. It is easily powdered and mixed with foods or blended into capsules; however, its taste leaves something to be desired. Usnea is most often tinctured, as it seems most effective in an alcohol solvent.

Uva ursi (*Arctostaphylos uva-ursi*)

PARTS USED: leaves, berries

BENEFITS: Uva ursi is a small, wiry shrub that hugs the earth. Its leatherlike leaves are infused to make a tea for kidney and bladder infections. It is an effective diuretic, astringent, and urinary antiseptic that cleans and heals urinary passages. It is also effective for cystitis, urethritis, kidney stones, and leukorrhea, and it can help put a stop to bed-wetting that results from lack of bladder tone or weak muscles.

SUGGESTED USES: Uva ursi is most effective as an infusion for inflammation and infection. A strong infusion mixed with cranberry juice can be helpful for bladder and kidney infections. However, a decoction will bring out a richer concentration of tannins and the plant's astringent properties.

Valerian (*Valeriana officinalis*)

PARTS USED: roots

BENEFITS: This is one of my favorite nerve tonics and muscle relaxants. It works very well for some people; a small percentage of people, however, find it irritating and overly stimulating. In those for whom it works, it is effective for insomnia, pain, restlessness, headaches, digestive problems due to nerves, and muscle spasms. Depending on the individual, the smell is either relished or deemed offensive. I rather love the odor, which reminds me of violets, or rich, sweet earth. Others may find that it smells too earthy, especially if the root is older.

SUGGESTED USES: Because the root is rich in volatile oils, it should be infused rather than decocted. Valerian is often tinctured or encapsulated rather than taken as tea because of its odor, though its taste is quite pleasant. Herbalists are in disagreement about whether the fresh or dried herb works better. I

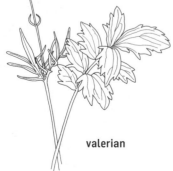

find it's a matter of personal preference. Without a doubt, it's better tasting and smelling when fresh, but I find the dried root works just as well as the fresh root. Cats love valerian root, also, even more than catnip. Sprinkle some in their bed or on the floor for some lively antics.

valerian

White oak (*Quercus alba*)

PART USED: the bark primarily, though the leaves and gall are also useful

BENEFITS: White oak is a huge, stately tree whose bark is a powerful astringent and disinfectant. The high tannin content in the bark, leaves, and gall makes the white oak especially useful for treating diarrhea, dysentery, and hemorrhoids, and it can be prepared as an astringent antiseptic wash for wounds, poison oak, and poison ivy. It is also used as a gargle for sore throats and tooth and gum infections, as a douche for leukorrhea, and as a wash or poultice for varicose veins.

SUGGESTED USES: The inner bark of the white oak is what is most often used, but the leaves and gall are also rich in tannins and very astringent. It is commonly made into a decoction for internal purposes, and an antiseptic liniment for external purposes. White oak bark also tinctures well and is often found in formulas for tooth/gum infections, sore throats, and skin infections such as poison oak and poison ivy.

Wild cherry (*Prunus serotina*)

PART USED: inner bark

BENEFITS: Wild cherry bark is one of the most reliable remedies for dry, hacking coughs. It is a pectoral expectorant, which means that it helps expel mucus from the lungs, and helps to relax and calm the pectoral muscles. It is one of the few herbs still included in the United States Pharmacopeia and can still be found in some commercial cough remedies.

It is also a digestive bitter that improves digestion and promotes healthy bowel function.

SUGGESTED USES: Wild cherry is a favorite herb to include in teas, syrups, and tinctures for coughs and colds. For dry, hacking coughs or spastic coughs that just won't stop, try blending wild cherry bark with valerian root. Made into a tea or tincture, this is an excellent combination that helps relax the muscles and expel deep-seated mucus.

Wild yam (*Dioscorea villosa*)

PARTS USED: roots

BENEFITS: Wild yam has a complex action on the body and is used for a variety of important purposes. It is a primary source material for steroid production and is a hormone precursor. It normalizes the function of the endocrine glands and aids in the normal function of the reproductive system of both sexes. It has been used to treat menstrual dysfunction, to stimulate the liver and digestion, and to increase fertility in women who are progesterone deficient. Wild yam also has nervine and antispasmodic properties, and it is an excellent remedy for soothing muscle cramps, colic, and uterine pain. It is also useful for relieving liver congestion and normalizing gallbladder function.

SUGGESTED USES: Use wild yam in formulas for the reproductive system of men and women. It can be made into teas, tinctures, and capsules.

CAUTION: This plant is listed on the United Plant Savers' "At-Risk" List (see page 120). It is seriously depleted in its natural habitat. Buy only from organically cultivated sources.

Witch hazel (*Hamamelis virginiana*)

PART USED: bark

BENEFITS: A North American shrub with the witchy habit of blooming in the winter long after all the other trees and shrubs have dropped their leaves, witch hazel is a well-known astringent tonic herb. The inner bark of the shrub is a potent pain reliever and astringent. It is thought to act on the venous system to stop bleeding and inflammation both internally and externally. It is particularly effective for intestinal bleeding, hemorrhoids, varicose veins, and diarrhea. It is also indicated to stop bleeding of the nose and lungs.

SUGGESTED USES: Witch hazel is often made into a tincture or liniment and used externally as an astringent, disinfectant wash. It also makes a good cleanser for troubled skin. Decocted as tea, it is used internally as an astringent for diarrhea and intestinal bleeding. It is still easy to find witch hazel extract in pharmacies, and even some grocery stores. Just make sure it is pure distilled witch hazel made from the bark of *Hamamelis virginiana*.

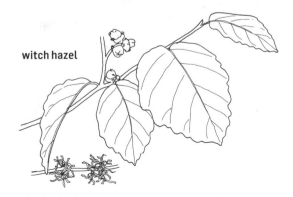

witch hazel

Yarrow (*Achillea millefolium* and related wild species)

PARTS USED: leaves, flowers

BENEFITS: Yarrow is one of our most versatile and healing plants, beloved and respected by those who use it. A beautiful roadside weed, yarrow is best recognized by its creamy white flowers that bloom in clusters atop a stalk throughout the summer months. Yarrow flowers and leaves are excellent diaphoretics (promote sweating). Diaphoretics like yarrow are often recommended to reduce a fever by helping a person produce sweat. Yarrow is also a very effective first aid remedy used to stop bleeding internally and externally. It can be applied externally as a poultice or wash or taken internally as a tea or tincture. It is also an effective remedy for menstrual and stomach cramps and muscle spasms. If that's not enough, yarrow also has beneficial effects on the heart and lungs.

SUGGESTED USES: Yarrow can be prepared as an infusion, tinctures well, and can be encapsulated. It does make a bitter infusion, so blend it with tastier herbs for use as a digestive aid and diaphoretic. The dried, powdered leaves and flowers are useful first aid items for disinfecting wounds and helping cuts stop bleeding. A pinch of the powder can be placed in the nose to stop a nosebleed.

Yellow dock (*Rumex crispus*)

PARTS USED: roots

BENEFITS: This abundant wild weed of fields, gardens, and roadsides is quite possibly one of the best herbs for the entire digestive system, including the liver. The large taproot is rich in anthraquinones, which have a laxative action. Though yellow dock root doesn't contain much iron itself, it aids in the assimilation and distribution of iron in our bodies, making it particularly useful for those with low iron. It is one of the best herbs for anemia and fatigue caused by low iron levels. Yellow dock is frequently included in formulas for women with PMS, and for both men and women with hormonal problems. The root is an excellent aid for sluggish digestion and constipation.

SUGGESTED USES: The chemical constituents are readily extracted by a water decoction and by alcohol. Yellow dock makes a somewhat bitter decoction, so it is best formulated with more flavorful herbs. The tincture is helpful for the liver, gallbladder, and digestion. It can be added to formulas for its laxative properties. It makes an iron-rich syrup; try adding other iron-rich herbs such as nettle, chickweed, and dandelion root and leaves.

CHAPTER FOUR

MAKING YOUR OWN FIRST AID KIT

You may find, as many others have, that herbs become a passion. Slowly but surely, they take over the entire house: first, it's only a small space in the bathroom closet; then, a cupboard in the kitchen is cleared; next, the entire basement is given over to your herbal wares; and suddenly, the cars are parked in the driveway because the garage is filled with bottles of odd-looking preparations. About this time, your family may be saying, "No more." But let's assume you're a long way from there and you just want to organize a small kit of useful herbal remedies.

WHAT DO I NEED?

TO MAKE AN HERBAL FIRST AID KIT, assess the needs of yourself and your family, and any situations that could arise requiring first aid. Do you have young children? What maladies are people in your family prone to?

A good kit consists of items that can be used for a variety of purposes. The most basic first aid kit will include the following:

- All-purpose/burn salve (burns, sunburns, cuts, wounds)
- Aloe vera gel (burns, sunburns, cuts, wounds)
- Antifungal salve (cuts, wounds)
- Cold care capsules (colds, sluggish digestion, infections)
- Echinacea tincture (boosting immunity, colds, flus, infections)
- Eucalyptus essential oil (congestion [added to steams], achy muscles, insect repellent, cuts and abrasions, warts, cold sores)
- Garlic oil (ear infections, parasites, colds)
- Green clay powder (splinters, disinfecting wounds, poultices for poison oak/ivy, skin infections)
- Kloss's Liniment (splinters and slivers, poison oak/ivy)
- Lavender essential oil (headaches, minor burns and sunburn, insect bites, congestion)
- Licorice root tincture (sore throats, bronchial inflammation, herpes simplex I and II)
- Garlic–Mullein Flower Oil (ear infections, pain)
- Peppermint essential oil (digestive problems, burns, mouthwash, stimulant)

- Rescue Remedy flower essence (trauma, both emotional and physical; can be used externally and internally for adults, children, and pets)
- St. John's wort salve (burns, sunburn, swellings, pain, bruises, achy muscles)
- St. John's Wort Oil (burns, pain, nerve damage, depression, anxiety)
- Tea tree essential oil (congestion [added to steams], achy muscles, insect repellent, cuts and abrasions, warts, cold sores, toothaches)
- Valerian tincture (pain, insomnia, stress and nervous tension, achy muscles)

Lots of herbs work well for minor emergencies. In addition to your favorite medicinal teas, stock an assortment of powdered herbs for different purposes; they are easy to mix for poultices and to encapsulate as needed.

Keep your herbal first aid kit in a place that's readily available to you and your family. Baskets, sewing boxes, small suitcases, travel pouches, cosmetic bags, and fishing tackle boxes make great containers for first aid kits. Be sure everything is clearly labeled so that others can use it. You might even wish to create a small first aid book that you keep near your remedies so that others can decipher what to use.

FIRST AID FROM THE KITCHEN

THOUGH NOT EVERYONE HAS A medicine chest full of medicinal herbs, everyone does have a kitchen. And, generally, that kitchen is filled with medicinal plants. Indeed, many of my favorite medicinal plants have sneaked into the household via the kitchen door, ushered in by the Mistress of Spices, their healing spirits camouflaged in culinary garb.

Most of your favorite kitchen herbs double as renowned healers, respected throughout the ages by various cultures. Many are still used in herbal remedies and even pharmaceutical preparations. Think of how we tend to associate the flavor of certain herbs with certain foods — basil with tomatoes, cloves with meat, horseradish with German food. In fact, these herbs were most often used with those foods for medicinal reasons, not for flavor. For example, basil aids with the digestion of the acids in tomatoes; cloves and other spices helped preserve meat in the days before refrigeration and prevented flies from laying eggs in it; and horseradish, long associated with rich, oily cuisine, stimulates the digestion of oil.

Following is a cornucopia of kitchen medicines. See chapter 3 for other useful and medicinal kitchen herbs and spices.

Basil

A favorite tonic for melancholy and low spirits, basil has antispasmodic properties that make it useful for headaches. It is commonly used to treat stress-induced insomnia and tension and nervous indigestion, and it is a well-known aphrodisiac.

Black pepper

Considered one of the great tonics in traditional Chinese medicine, black pepper is warming, energizing, and stimulating. It is indicated for slow circulation, poor digestion, and "cold type" problems such as flus, coughs, and colds. Some people find it an irritant. Jethro Kloss, a famous herbalist of the early 1900s, publicized it as a toxic substance. However, most people tolerate it well.

Cardamom

With a divinely sensual flavor, cardamom, which belongs to the same family as ginger, stimulates the mind and arouses the senses. It has long been considered an aphrodisiac, in part because of its irresistible flavor. In Ayurvedic medicine, cardamom is considered one of the best digestive aids. It is often combined as an anticatarrhal (combating inflammation of the mucous membranes) in formulas for the lungs.

Chives

Chives are similar to garlic, though not as potent, so people sensitive to garlic can often enjoy chives' medicinal and culinary offerings. Like garlic, chives have antiseptic properties, and they also help in the digestion of rich foods and protect the respiratory system.

Cinnamon

Highly valued in traditional Chinese medicine as a warming and stimulating herb, cinnamon is used to boost vitality, stimulate circulation, and clear congestion. It is a well-respected digestive aid, has powerful antiseptic actions as well, and is indicated for poor digestion, colds, and flus. With its pleasingly spicy flavor, cinnamon is often used in medicinal formulas to mask the flavor of less tasty herbs.

Cloves

Clove oil is most famous as an analgesic for toothaches, but the entire clove bud, powdered and applied directly to the gum, is as effective. Aside from its analgesic properties, clove is stimulating, warming, and uplifting. It is used for sluggish digestion and nausea.

Dill

Dill is one of the most famous of traditional English remedies for infant colic, extolled in medicinal writings and nursery songs alike. Dill's warming and comforting qualities are indicated for gas and colicky digestion. Dill is also an old folk remedy for hiccups.

Horseradish

What better natural remedy is there for sinus congestion and head colds? This is my number one favorite. The root is rich in minerals, including silica, and in vitamins, including vitamin C. Its warming antiseptic properties make it the herb of choice for asthma, catarrh, and lung infections. Horseradish is also prized as a digestive aid and is especially useful as a complement to heavy, hard-to-digest meals.

Marjoram and oregano

Calming and soothing herbs, both marjoram and oregano are used for nervousness, irritability, and insomnia due to tension and anxiety. They are great to drink as a tea — either in combination or singly — when you're feeling edgy, or to calm butterflies in the stomach. These delicious herbs also have antispasmodic properties that can be used advantageously for digestive and muscular spasms.

Parsley

This superb garnish should never be left slighted on the side of a platter. It may be, in fact, the most nourishing item on your dinner plate. High in iron, beta-carotene, and chlorophyll, parsley is used to treat iron-poor blood, anemia, and fatigue. It will enhance immunity and is indicated when you are prone to infections. A primary herb for bladder and kidney problems, it is a safe, effective diuretic. Parsley is used for helping to dry up a mother's milk during the weaning process and is effective as a poultice for mastitis or swollen, enlarged breasts. Because of this, you should not use parsley in any quantities when nursing, as it may slow the flow of milk.

Rocket (Arugula)

Imagine my delight when I discovered that arugula, my favorite salad green, was a famous sexual stimulant and tonic. I'm not sure whether to indulge more or be more temperate in my servings.

Thyme

This is the best herb we have for stimulating the thymus, a major gland of the immune system. Thyme is a great pick-me-up when you have low energy. Its antispasmodic properties are useful for lung problems and for convulsive coughs, such as whooping cough. It's an excellent remedy for sore throats (combined with sage), head colds (combined with horseradish), and stiffness related to chills. Thyme also helps stimulate the body's natural defenses and, combined with echinacea, boosts the immune system.

Turmeric

This is one of the best herbs for immune health and is often overlooked because of the huge popularity of echinacea. But, for centuries, it has upheld its reputation for its immune-enhancing properties and is highly regarded for its anti-tumor and antibiotic activities. In East Indian medicine, it is valued as a blood purifier and metabolic tonic. It is used to regulate the menstrual cycle and relieve cramps, reduce fevers, improve poor circulation, and relieve skin disorders. It is highly valued as a first aid treatment for boils, burns, strains, swelling, and bruises.

CHAPTER FIVE

SIMPLE & EFFECTIVE HOME REMEDIES

In the past, common, everyday ailments were treated either by someone in the family or by the local healer or herbalist. Many of these problems respond well to herbal treatment. I have included several common maladies here, along with favorite suggestions and time-tested recipes for effective herbal medicines.

If your situation does not respond to these safe and simple suggestions within an appropriate time frame, or if the symptoms get progressively worse, seek the help of a health care professional, ideally one knowledgeable about natural remedies. When dealing with life-threatening illnesses, you should, of course, seek professional medical help as quickly as possible. But most of the health issues we deal with daily don't require expensive pharmaceuticals or a doctor's visit.

ATHLETE'S FOOT

ATHLETE'S FOOT IS A fungal infection of the feet. Often itchy, it can spread to the hands. In dealing with athlete's foot, it is important to keep your feet dry and your socks clean, and to go shoeless or to wear sandals as much as possible to air your feet.

What to Do

Tea tree essential oil, with its potent antifungal properties, can be helpful. Sprinkle the essential oil directly on the infected area, and/or soak your feet several times a week in a hot footbath with tea tree and chaparral essential oils added to it. In addition, try the following remedies.

Antifungal Salve

This salve was created for athlete's foot and works especially well for dry or chapped areas, lesions, and cracks. I have used it successfully for other fungal infections, as well as for mange on animals. If you can't find organically grown goldenseal, just omit it from this formula.

- 2 parts black walnut hulls
- 2 parts chaparral
- 1 part echinacea
- 1 part goldenseal (organically cultivated)
- 1 part myrrh
  a few drops of cajeput or tea tree essential oil

Use the herbs to prepare a salve, following the instructions on page 20. Apply twice daily, in the morning and evening.

Antifungal Powder

This is an effective powder that is also simple to make. If you can't find organically grown goldenseal, eliminate it from this recipe.

- ½ cup white cosmetic-grade clay (or arrowroot powder)
- 1 tablespoon black walnut hulls
- 1 tablespoon chaparral powder
- 1 teaspoon goldenseal (organically cultivated)
- 1 teaspoon tea tree essential oil

Combine the clay, black walnut hulls, chaparral, and goldenseal. Add the tea tree essential oil and mix well. Let dry; store in a shaker bottle. Apply to the feet once or twice daily. Please note: black walnut will stain the feet black but only for a few days.

BURNS

BURNS CAN RESULT FROM fire, heat, overexposure to sunlight, or chemicals. First- and second-degree burns can generally be treated effectively at home, but you must be certain to keep the area clean to avoid infection. If infection should occur, seek medical advice. Always seek medical attention for third-degree burns.

What to Do

To treat a burn, first cool the area, thus "putting out the fire." Immerse the area in ice water or apply a compress of diluted apple cider vinegar for at least a half hour. Next, choose one or more of the following treatments:

- Add 2 to 3 drops of peppermint essential oil to ¼ cup of honey for a cooling disinfectant poultice, and apply to the burn.
- Apply aloe vera gel, which is cooling, disinfectant, and healing.
- Take valerian tincture (see pages 22–23) internally to alleviate pain.
- For burns from hot foods on the roof of the mouth, take pill balls made with slippery elm and honey (see the instructions on pages 17–18) to heal the burn and lessen the pain.
- Prepare and apply St. John's Wort Salve.

St. John's Wort Salve

St. John's Wort Salve or St. John's Wort Oil (see page 63) applied topically are especially helpful for healing burns and any damaged nerve endings. This is an excellent, all-purpose salve that can also be used for rashes, cuts, and wounds of all types.

> 1 part calendula flowers
> 1 part comfrey leaf
> 1 part St. John's wort (leaves and flowers)

Use the herbs to prepare a salve, following the instructions on page 20. Apply to the affected area two or three times daily.

COLDS AND FLUS

COLDS AND FLUS ARE viral infections of the upper respiratory tract, often involving the throat, eyes, nose, and head. Bed rest is always recommended to treat these illnesses. Thankfully, there are many inexpensive treatments readily available.

What to Do

Eat lightly, avoiding all dairy products and anything else that will cause more mucus to accumulate in the system, such as sugar — including orange juice. Foods should be simple and warming. Hot broth is perfect for colds, and you can add medicinal herbs such as astragalus and echinacea to it. And, of course, eat lots of onions and garlic, nature's best remedies for colds and flus. The following may also be helpful:

- Cook with traditional curry blends, which are a mix of medicinal herbs, including turmeric and cayenne, that stimulate and activate the immune system. Sauté onion slices and whole cloves of garlic with lots of curry. It not only tastes divine but clears the sinuses, while effectively fighting the cold or flu virus.
- Drink several cups a day of tea made with yarrow, peppermint, and elder. This is an old Gypsy formula that is very effective for helping sweat out a cold or flu.
- Make hot ginger tea with freshly grated ginger, honey, and lemon. This is one of the tastiest things you can take for a cold. For an extra punch, I'll sprinkle a bit of cayenne in

the tea. Drinking several cups of this daily will help sweat out a cold.

- Elderberry syrup is another tasty cold and flu remedy, and it's one of the most effective remedies you can make. Elderberries contain broad-spectrum antiviral properties and are able to fight off many different types of viruses. You can make elderberry syrup using either fresh or dried berries, following the instructions on page 15.
- Make your own echinacea tincture (see pages 22–23 for instructions) before the cold season starts. To ward off a cold, take ½ teaspoon of the tincture every half hour at the first sign of symptoms. If you already have a cold, take 1 teaspoon of the tincture every 2 hours.

Fire Cider

This is another of my favorite remedies that is effective, easy to make, and tasty, but not for the weak of heart. Make a batch before the cold season starts.

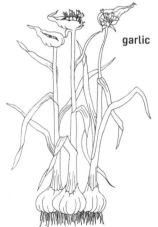

garlic

1 quart apple cider vinegar
¼ cup grated fresh horseradish
1 onion, chopped
1 head of garlic, peeled and chopped

(continued on next page)

2   tablespoons powdered turmeric
    cayenne powder
1   cup honey (more or less to taste)

Combine the vinegar, horseradish, onion, garlic, turmeric, and a pinch or two of cayenne. Cover and let sit in a warm place for 3–4 weeks. Strain the mixture, add the honey, and rebottle. Refrigerate. Take 1–2 tablespoons at the first sign of a cold and continue throughout the day (approximately every 2–3 hours) until the symptoms subside.

CONJUNCTIVITIS

A HIGHLY CONTAGIOUS inflammation of the eye, conjunctivitis causes the eyes to get red, swollen, and itchy. The tendency is to rub the itchy eye and then, unthinkingly, rub the other eye, thereby transferring the infection. Children often pass conjunctivitis among themselves.

What to Do

The immune system is often compromised in cases of conjunctivitis; use echinacea to boost natural immunity. Administer ½ to 1 teaspoon every hour, decreasing the dosage as symptoms subside.

For severe itching, pain, and irritation, make a tea using equal amounts of lemon balm, lavender, and chamomile; drink several cups a day. Augment the relaxing and pain-relieving properties of the tea with 1 teaspoon of valerian tincture (see pages 22–23) several times daily.

Eyewash

Use this eyewash to treat conjunctivitis without antibiotics. Be sure to strain the liquid well; you don't want any herb particles to get into the eyes. If you prefer, mix the herbs into a paste with a small amount of warm water, and then spread the paste on a piece of gauze and apply as a poultice over the eyes.

> 1 tablespoon comfrey root powder
> 1 teaspoon goldenseal root powder (organically cultivated)
> 1 cup boiling water

Combine the herbs, and pour the boiling water over them. Strain well through two or three layers of muslin, or a fine coffee filter. Allow the liquid to cool to room temperature. Using an eyecup or eye dropper, wash the eyes several times a day with the eyewash. Continue until symptoms subside, usually within 4–5 days.

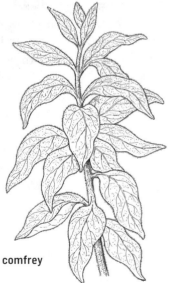

comfrey

CONSTIPATION

INFREQUENT OR DIFFICULT bowel movements are best treated with herbs. We won't get into a discussion here of what is considered "infrequent"; however, if you don't have a regular bowel movement at least once a day, consider constipation a problem. If constipation is chronic, consult a holistic health care practitioner.

What to Do

It's tempting for herbalists to treat this situation with heroic herbs in much the same manner that allopathic medicine would. Cascara sagrada and senna, for example, are excellent laxatives and will get things moving. However, they will also create dependencies when used too often or too strongly, so we can't rely on them. Instead, focus on the following:

Contributing factors. The first step to addressing constipation is to eliminate factors that contribute to it. Diet is important; cheese, pasta, and bread are just a few of the foods that frequently cause constipation in people with sluggish bowels. Other contributors include stress and tension, lack of exercise, and inadequate hydration. Drink 6 to 8 cups of pure water daily if constipation is a problem.

Bulking up. A good daily remedy is a mixture of 1 tablespoon each of ground psyllium seeds and ground flaxseed. Add the ground seeds to cereal, salads, or other foods. You must drink several cups of water daily when using these seeds.

Magnesium. Another easy and simple remedy for relieving constipation is to take a magnesium supplement. Magnesium is relaxing and calming to the muscles. Begin by taking the dosage recommended by the supplement label, and increase just until bowel movements become soft (not loose) and regular.

Liver health. You can also try using a formula that supports digestion and liver health. I've found yellow dock root to be excellent for constipation, without any of the dependency issues. Mix 2 parts yellow dock root with 1 part dandelion root and 1 part licorice root, and prepare as a tea. Drink 3 cups of this daily. In addition, a tincture made from this formula may be used for difficult cases.

Triphala. One of the absolute best herbal remedies for people who suffer from long-term sluggish digestion and constipation is an Ayurvedic formula called triphala. Triphala is probably the most widely used formula in the world for digestive issues. It is mild and effective and doesn't create dependency. It is commonly available in herb and natural food stores.

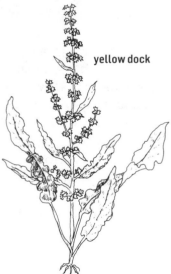

yellow dock

CUTS AND WOUNDS

LARGE OR DEEP WOUNDS will need medical attention, but you can treat minor cuts, lesions, scrapes, and bites at home.

What to Do

Wash any cuts with an antiseptic solution, such as witch hazel extract with tea tree essential oil (use 6 to 8 drops of tea tree essential oil per cup of witch hazel). If necessary, disinfect the area with Kloss's Liniment (see page 93).

To stop bleeding, apply a poultice or compress of yarrow (the leaf and flower both work) and/or shepherd's purse and yarrow. Keep the poultice in place until the wound stops bleeding. Believe it or not, clean cobwebs will also stop bleeding.

If the wound contains a splinter, soak it in water and Epsom salts, or apply a thick clay pack (of green or red clay) directly to the spot. Leave it on for several hours; change once or twice during the day. Once the splinter has been drawn out, disinfect the area with Kloss's Liniment, a lavender wash, or a similar remedy.

When the wound has been cleaned and the area disinfected, apply St. John's Wort Salve (see page 85) and wrap the area in a gauze bandage or cotton flannel cloth. If the cut is painful, take lemon balm, valerian, and chamomile tea or tincture.

Several types of poultices may also be helpful. Depending on the seriousness of the wound, apply one of these:

- A clay poultice if the wound is quite large, with the possibility of infection
- A plantain poultice directly to the wound to stop bleeding and prevent infection
- A comfrey poultice to encourage healing of torn tissue and to soothe pain and inflammation

Kloss's Liniment

This liniment, from the famous herb doctor Jethro Kloss, is useful for inflammation of the muscles, though I use it primarily as a disinfectant. If organically grown goldenseal isn't available, substitute chaparral or Oregon grape root.

1 ounce echinacea powder
1 ounce goldenseal powder (organically cultivated)
1 ounce myrrh powder
¼ ounce cayenne powder
1 pint rubbing alcohol

Mix the herbs. Prepare as a tincture in the rubbing alcohol, following the instructions on pages 22–23. Clearly label the container FOR EXTERNAL USE ONLY.

Goldenseal Salve

This salve is excellent when an astringent, disinfectant action is needed. It also serves as an emollient. If organically grown goldenseal is not available, substitute chaparral.

> 1 part goldenseal (organically cultivated)
> 1 part myrrh gum

Combine the herbs and prepare as a salve, following the instructions on page 20.

DIARRHEA

ONE OF THE MOST COMMON ailments to afflict humankind, diarrhea is characterized by loose, watery bowel movements. This problem can be caused by factors such as infection, parasites, unbalanced diet, and even stress. While everyone experiences diarrhea from time to time, if you have chronic diarrhea, you should consult a holistic health care practitioner or a physician.

What to Do

Blackberry root tincture (see pages 21–23) is my favorite remedy for diarrhea. At the first signs of diarrhea, take ½ teaspoon of the tincture every half hour until symptoms subside.

If blackberry root is not available, any strong astringent such as white oak bark, witch hazel bark (not the extract sold in pharmacies), or raspberry leaf will do. Black tea also works in a pinch.

At the same time that you're trying to dry things up, use teas or tinctures of mucilaginous herbs such as marsh mallow or licorice to soothe irritated bowels. For example, try a tea made with two parts blackberry root and one part licorice root; drink 3 to 4 cups daily. If the diarrhea is persistent, add chaparral or goldenseal to the tea. Combine any of these herbs with oatmeal porridge for a soothing, edible remedy.

It is essential to drink sufficient quantities of water when you're experiencing diarrhea; it is very easy to become dehydrated. Squeezing the juice of a fresh lemon into the water is even better. Be especially mindful of hydration with small children, and ensure that their liquid intake is sufficient (several cups of water a day in addition to their medicinal tea).

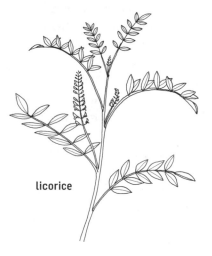

licorice

EARACHE

EARACHES ARE INFECTIONS of the inner or outer ear signified by pain, redness, and sometimes itchiness around the outer ear. Mild earaches can be readily treated at home. If the pain gets severe or is prolonged, consult a holistic health care provider or a physician.

What to Do

Hot onion packs are an old-fashioned remedy that can really work. Sauté onions until soft, and then wrap the onions in a flannel cloth and apply directly to both ears (one at a time, if desired). Reheat the onions as needed. Leave the hot onion pack on for 30–45 minutes, and longer if possible.

If the ear still hurts, heat some salt in a cast-iron skillet, and when it is too hot to touch, pour it onto a dishcloth or cotton cloth. Fold carefully, being sure not to burn yourself. Using more towels to protect against the heat, place the pack against the ear for at least 30 minutes. Treat both ears, as the ear canals are connected, and the infection can easily move back and forth. Hot salt packs work best if there is a lot of moisture and congestion in the ears. In addition to the hot packs, you can try infection-fighting oil treatments; see the recipe for garlic-mullein oil on page 97.

Earaches are generally accompanied by a cold or flu. Treat the related symptoms, and eliminate foods that may be congesting to the eardrums, such as dairy, sugar, and citrus products (with the exception of lemons and grapefruit). And take ½ to 1 teaspoon of echinacea tincture (see pages 22–23) several times a day to activate the immune system.

Treating Swimmer's Ear

Swimmer's ear is an ear infection caused by water in the eardrum. It doesn't respond well to oil applications; in fact, oil treatments will often make it worse. Instead, combine several drops of tea tree or lavender essential oil with ¼ cup of rubbing alcohol. Shake well. Using a dropper, apply several drops in each ear. Massage the outer ear. Repeat several times daily, until symptoms subside. Hot salt packs (see facing page) are often helpful for swimmer's ear.

Garlic–Mullein Flower Oil

This is a wonderful remedy for ear infections that relieves the pain and helps eliminate the infection. St. John's Wort Oil (see recipe on page 63) is often added to this blend to enhance its effectiveness. The flowers of mullein are often difficult to purchase, so gather some in the summer and fall when the plant is in bloom.

- 2–3 tablespoons chopped garlic
- 2–3 tablespoons mullein flowers
  virgin olive oil
- 2–3 tablespoons St. John's Wort Oil (optional)

Combine the garlic and mullein, and infuse in the olive oil, following the instructions on page 12. Add the St. John's Wort Oil, if you're using it. Warm the mixture only to body temperature and apply 3–4 drops in each ear. Massage the outer ear and around the base of the ear. Repeat several times daily, until symptoms subside.

FEVER

ANY TEMPERATURE OVER 98.6°F (37°C) is considered a fever. Fever is the immune system's natural defense for stopping infection and disease. However, out-of-control fevers can be devastating. A fever over 104°F (40°C) should receive immediate attention from your health care provider; do not wait for a fever to climb this high before taking action, especially with children.

What to Do

For low fevers, make a big pot of ginger-lemon tea, or a combination of peppermint, elder, and yarrow, and drink several hot, steaming cups. Wrap up in blankets and sweat out the infection.

To relieve headache and lower a fever, wrap the forehead and feet with washcloths dipped in cold water, with a few drops of lavender essential oil added to it. (Or attempt a whole-body cold wrap; see page 9.) And take ½ to 1 teaspoon of echinacea tincture several times daily to boost the immune system.

Drink lots of fluids during a fever, and avoid foods and drinks that are dehydrating (coffee, black tea, soda). If the patient cannot tolerate liquids, or the fever is rising rapidly, a catnip enema can be excellent for lowering the fever and hydrating the system, especially in children. You will need an appropriate-size enema bag with a pressure regulator on the tubing. Don't attempt an enema without expert guidance; consult with your health care provider if necessary.

Cold Wraps

Cold (or tepid) sheet wraps are one of the best techniques for lowering fever, hydrating the system, and improving circulation. Cold wraps are administered in bed, which will need to be protected with plastic sheeting. Soak a bedsheet in a large pan of cold or tepid water. Essential oils such as lavender, eucalyptus, tea tree, cajeput, pine, or cedar can be added to the water or sprinkled on the sheet to enhance the therapeutic value of the wrap. Wring out the sheet, and then place it on the plastic sheeting. Instruct the patient to lie down in the middle of the sheet. Wrap it snugly around him or her, from toes to neck, leaving only the head protruding. Place a tepid, damp cloth on the forehead.

This treatment should be administered for 15 to 20 minutes only. Do not let the person get chilled; be sure the temperature of the room is warm. After the wrap, serve a large cup of warm ginger tea, and put the patient directly into a warm, comfy bed.

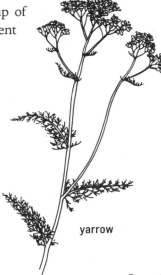

yarrow

HEARTBURN

THIS UNPLEASANT BURNING sensation behind the breastbone — sometimes accompanied by a sulfurlike flavor in the mouth — is caused by spasms and irritation in the esophagus or upper stomach. Heartburn is a sure sign that you are offending your stomach in some manner. Stress, too much food, and a too-rich diet are common causes of heartburn.

What to Do

The best herbs to use for heartburn are those that calm the nervous system and are good for digestive nervousness, such as chamomile, hops, and lemon balm. Mucilaginous herbs such as marsh mallow and licorice root, which soothe an irritated stomach lining, are also helpful.

Prepare an infusion (see pages 12–13) of 2 parts lemon balm, 1 part chamomile, and 1 part licorice, and drink a cup ½ hour before and after meals to prevent heartburn. To aid digestion, take hops tincture and/or a digestive bitter — such as Urban Moonshine's bitters or Swedish bitters, or your own digestive bitter tincture using the recipe on page 105 — with every meal.

Peppermint tea is often very helpful as a preventive; drink before and after meals. Try adding a drop or two of peppermint essential oil to water and drinking small sips during the meal.

Relax during and after meals. Try deep breathing, offering prayer before your meal, and chewing slowly, counting your chews. And don't eat when you're upset; take a walk instead.

HEADACHES

HEADACHES, TYPIFIED BY THROBBING or dull pain in the head, have a variety of causes, ranging from eating too much and too fast to emotional factors. They are a sure sign that things are "not okay," at least for the moment.

What to Do

Most headaches respond well to simple care. Try any or all of these treatments:

Lavender bath. Baths are soothing, and lavender essential oil enhances the calming effect. If a full bath is not possible, use lavender essential oil in a hot herbal footbath. Rubbing the shoulders while soaking the feet is often helpful in alleviating a headache. You may also wrap the head in a cool cloth sprinkled with lavender essential oil.

Valerian tincture. Used for stress-related headaches, valerian tincture (see pages 22–23) is extremely effective. Take ¼ teaspoon of the tincture every half hour until symptoms subside.

Salted plums and miso soup. If the headache is of the vascular type caused by a rich diet, too much sugar, or a highly charged emotional state, try eating Japanese salted plums or a cup of miso soup. This alkalizes the blood quickly, changing the pH, and will often diminish the headache.

Headache Tea

Different people respond to different headache remedies. This is one of my favorite combinations; it also makes a great tincture for headaches and migraines alike. Headache Tea is even more effective if used in conjunction with a hot lavender bath.

> 2 parts lemon balm
> 1 part feverfew
> 1 part lavender
> 1 part California poppy
>   (seeds, leaves, and flowers; optional)

Mix the herbs. Prepare as a tea, following the directions on page 11. Drink ¼ cup every half hour.

Treating Migraines

MIGRAINES ARE excruciatingly painful, recurring, and often difficult to treat because there are so many underlying causes. Food allergies, hormonal imbalances, light or the lack of it, and stress are only a few of the factors that can trigger a migraine. Trying to get to the source(s) of what causes the migraines is the key to developing an effective treatment program.

As a preventive, feverfew often works for people for whom nothing else has worked. However, it must be used over a period of at least 3 months before you can determine whether it works. If you grow feverfew, eat a leaf or two daily. It can also be dried and used in tea; drink a cup or two daily. I recommend tincturing this herb with lavender (see pages 21–23); take 1 teaspoon daily as a preventive. Feverfew is not recommended for use during pregnancy.

When you feel a migraine coming on, mix ½ teaspoon of guarana with two packages of Alacer's Emergen-C (found in natural food stores), and drink. Repeat if necessary. If guarana is not available, take a large dose of coffee. It may keep you up, but often it averts the headache.

When you feel a migraine coming on, a tincture of the herbs used in Headache Tea (see page 102) can be helpful. And drink Headache Tea daily as a migraine preventive.

INDIGESTION AND POOR DIGESTION

THE INABILITY TO DIGEST foods creates sluggish elimination, gas, and poor assimilation of nutrients. Poor digestion and pain and gas in the abdomen are usually a result of poor eating habits, low-quality food, and stress. Therefore, indigestion responds well to lifestyle changes. Low levels of digestive enzymes and intestinal flora can also cause digestive problems.

What to Do

Before changing your diet or adding supplements and herbs, try these simple suggestions:

- Say a prayer before your meal; honor the food that you're about to eat.
- Chew slowly and thoughtfully. If engaging in conversation, keep your voice quiet and conversation peaceful.

- Don't rush through your meal. Enjoy it as if it were your last one.
- Don't drink cold fluids with your meal; in fact, it's best not to drink immediately before or after a meal. If you must drink with your meals, drink liquid at room temperature. It is best not to drink coffee, black tea, or sodas with meals.
- Be careful what foods you combine at meals. Combining carbohydrates and protein ensures gas and putrefaction in the system. Educate yourself about food combinations that aid digestion.

In addition to changing your habits:
- Drink a cup of peppermint and chamomile tea ½ hour before and after meals.
- Buy a ready-made digestive bitter such as Urban Moonshine's bitters or Swedish bitters (available at health food stores), or make your own digestive bitter tincture (see the recipe on page 105). Take a dose with every meal.
- Add fresh ginger and cayenne to your food, or drink a warm tea made with them if you have slow digestion.
- Take papaya enzymes with meals to aid digestion.
- Take a daily supplement of acidophilus. It restores weak intestinal flora and is readily available at natural food stores.
- Combine carminative seeds to chew at and between meals. Dill, cardamom, anise, fennel, and cumin are all very helpful for reducing gas and bloated stomachs.

Digestive Bitter Tincture

2 parts fennel
1 part artichoke leaf
1 part dandelion root
1 part motherwort
½ part ginger

Mix the herbs and prepare as a tincture, following the instructions on pages 22–23. Take ½–1 teaspoon before and after meals.

JET LAG

WHEN YOU TRAVEL through one or more time zones in a day, your body is sometimes unable to adjust. Its hormone levels and biorhythms are disturbed, resulting in a feeling of disorientation, sometimes nausea, and depression. Flying can be stressful on its own, but it also subjects travelers to recycled air, germs, dehydration, and the like. People who fly often find themselves with compromised immune systems and more prone to illness, stress, and depression.

What to Do

Following are some tips for staying healthy in the air:

- Take Alacer's Emergenc-C (2,000 mg) daily for several days before traveling.
- Take two capsules (400 to 500 mg each) of Siberian ginseng three times daily for several days before traveling.

- Make a tincture of ginkgo, hawthorn, and St. John's wort and take ½–1 teaspoon three times a day for several days before flying. This is one of my personal favorites for preventing jet lag.
- Drink plenty of water when flying. I usually pack an empty quart bottle that I can fill once I'm through the security gates. They do serve water on planes, but it's never enough. Drink several quarts while you're in the air. It may mean frequent trips to the restroom, but that's a good excuse to exercise on the plane.
- Carry a spritzer bottle of water with Rescue Remedy and a few drops of lavender essential oil added. I always fly with this, and no one ever seems to mind when I freshen the stale air in the plane with a few sprays.
- Take echinacea tincture for a few days before and after flying if your immune system is stressed and you're feeling particularly vulnerable to illness.
- Pack kava tincture and take it frequently throughout your travels if you find traveling to be stressful. You'll be noticeably less stressed, and perhaps you'll even enjoy a warm, sweet feeling of euphoria.

INSOMNIA

SLEEPLESSNESS OR RESTLESS sleep is a big problem for someone who is already anxious or stressed. Not only does lack of sleep leave us worn out and tired, it can also agitate stress and anxiety, provoking a chronic sense of distress and depletion.

Sleep refuels us not just physically and energetically but also psychologically. The body needs sleep in order to dream. Our dreams are important to our health and psyche, whether or not we remember them.

What to Do

Sometimes people are unable to sleep because of stimulating food or drink consumed earlier in the day. If you're having trouble sleeping, eliminate or reduce any stimulants in your diet; if you must have them to get your day going, don't have any after 10 a.m. These would include coffee, black tea, green tea, and stimulating herbs such as ginseng, rhodiola, and yerba mate. Also eliminate or reduce any sugar, chocolate, and red wine in the evening, all of which can be stimulating.

Other helpful aids for good sleep include the following:

St. John's wort. My favorite solution for insomnia is St. John's wort — it works almost every time. Take ½ teaspoon of St. John's wort tincture three times daily for 5 days, stop for 2 days, and repeat the cycle until you're able to sleep peacefully.

Nervines. Throughout the day, drink a good nervine tea such as a blend of lemon balm, chamomile, and passionflower, stopping 3 hours before bedtime. Or take 1 teaspoon of a combination hops-and-valerian tincture each hour for 2 to 3 hours before bedtime. Passionflower and skullcap is another combination that works especially well for those whose brains just won't slow down. For people who can't sleep because of anxiety, try kava tincture before bedtime.

Baths or walks. Just before bed, take either a warm lavender bath or an invigorating walk. If it is possible to walk barefoot on a grassy area, do so. It connects you to the electromagnetic forces of the earth. Curl up in bed following your bath or walk. You'll usually go right to sleep.

LARYNGITIS AND SORE THROAT

THOUGH SORE THROATS and laryngitis are not technically the same, they respond to the same treatments. Laryngitis is an inflammation of the throat, resulting in hoarseness and an occasional sore throat. Laryngitis is generally a result of an infection or stressed vocal cords. Sore throats are usually a result of infection but don't necessarily result in laryngitis.

What to Do

The best and surest cure for laryngitis is to rest the voice. Several herbal companies make excellent throat sprays incorporating echinacea, licorice, slippery elm, and other herbs specific to soothing irritated vocal cords. Make your own by brewing a triple-strength tea of licorice, echinacea, and sage (3 teaspoons of herb per cup), and add a few drops of tea tree, peppermint, or eucalyptus essential oil to it. Put the mix in a mister or spray bottle and squirt it into the back of the throat as needed.

Sage is often helpful for relieving sore throats and laryngitis. Prepare it as an infusion (see pages 12–13), and use as both a tea and a gargle.

Throat Soother Tea

This tea strengthens the voice and soothes throat irritation.

- 2 parts licorice root
- 1 part cinnamon
- 1 part echinacea
- 1 part marsh mallow root
- ⅛ part ginger

Mix the herbs and prepare as a decoction, following the instructions on page 13. Drink several cups of tea a day.

Cough Be Gone & Sore Throat Syrup

This syrup for sore and inflamed throats is much tastier than my Sore Throat Gargle. (See the recipe on page 110.)

- 4 parts fennel seeds
- 2 parts licorice root
- 2 parts marsh mallow root
- 2 parts valerian
- 2 parts wild cherry bark
- 1 part cinnamon bark
- ½ part gingerroot
- ⅛ part orange peel

Mix the herbs and prepare as a syrup, following the instructions on page 14. Take 1–2 teaspoons every hour or two throughout the day, or use whenever a bout of coughing starts up.

Sore Throat Gargle

This is my favorite gargle for sore throats and laryngitis; however, I'm the first to admit that it's not my tastiest recipe.

- 1 cup apple cider vinegar
- 1 cup strong sage tea (triple strength)
- 2–3 tablespoons salt
   pinch of cayenne

Combine all the ingredients and shake to mix. Gargle with this mixture frequently throughout the day.

Throat Balls

This tasty herbal candy is excellent for sore throats and even for strep throat. If organically grown goldenseal is unavailable, substitute Oregon grape root.

- 1 part carob powder
- 1 part licorice root powder
- 1 part marsh mallow powder
- ½ part echinacea powder
- ¼ part goldenseal powder (organically cultivated)
   a few drops of peppermint essential oil

Use the herbs and essential oil to make a batch of herbal candy, following the instructions on page 16. Take one marble-sized ball three to four times daily.

POISON OAK AND POISON IVY

THESE BEAUTIFUL WOODLAND vines can cause a nasty hot, itchy rash. This contact dermatitis can get quite severe in sensitive people.

What to Do

I've used Kloss's Liniment (page 93) successfully for stopping the itch and spread of poison oak and ivy. Dilute it with water or witch hazel extract so that it stings but doesn't burn. Keep the bottle handy and apply frequently throughout the day.

In areas where it's not possible to use the liniment (genitals and eyes), use plain unsweetened yogurt. Yogurt is cooling, drying, and disinfecting. Cover the affected area and let dry.

Assist the body in healing by taking echinacea tincture (see pages 21–23) throughout the day. Since the rash produces a "hot" condition in the body, it is important to use cooling herbs to help with the symptoms. Cleavers, chickweed, burdock, and

Coping with Poison Oak and Poison Ivy

For the irritation, which at times can be unbearable, take frequent doses of kava and/or valerian tincture (½ teaspoon of the tincture every 2 hours). If you tend to scratch the rash at night, which is common, do what parents do to infants: cover the hands with socks at night.

dandelion are all recommended. Make a tea with a combination of these herbs, and drink several cups a day.

Along similar lines, avoid spicy foods, as they will agitate the heat condition and make the itch worse. Though it's tempting to take a hot bath or shower that will make the rash feel better temporarily, heat will likely agitate the condition in the long run. Bathe only in tepid water.

Ocean water is one of the most healing treatments for these rashes. If you live near the sea, bathe in it daily. Or simulate the ocean waters in your tub: add kelp, baking soda, and sea salt to the tub, and bathe in cool water only. A drop or two of peppermint essential oil (no more or you'll be jumping out of that tub before you get all the way in it!) will help cool the rash and give temporary relief from the burning.

Itch Relief Remedy

This is my favorite remedy for poison oak or ivy. Store this wonderful healing cream in a glass container with a tight-fitting lid. If it dries out, reconstitute by adding water.

>   1   cup green volcanic clay powder
>   water or witch hazel extract
>   2   tablespoons salt
> 4–6   drops peppermint essential oil

Mix the clay with enough water or witch hazel extract to make a creamy paste. Add the salt and several drops of the peppermint essential oil; the paste should smell strong and feel cooling to the skin. Spread directly on the affected area and leave on until the paste is completely dry. To rinse off, soak a washcloth in water or witch hazel extract and rub gently. Don't scrub the skin.

TOOTHACHE

WHO HASN'T HAD one of these? A toothache can be caused by stress or anxiety, but it is generally caused by bacteria infecting the tissue at the base of the tooth. The pain is the irritated nerve sending a signal that something is awry.

What to Do

Make an appointment to see a good dentist. In the meantime, try any of the following:

- You can alleviate and often cure a toothache by applying poultices of herbs directly to the site of infection.
- Clove oil applied topically is an effective analgesic for toothaches, helping to relieve the pain.
- Valerian, if taken in sufficiently high dosages (½ teaspoon of the tincture every half hour), will also help lessen the pain.
- Spilanthes, too, has antiseptic and analgesic properties and is my favorite remedy for easing the pain of toothaches. Make a mouth rinse of spilanthes and use it frequently. Employed on a regular basis, it will also help with long-term tooth and gum health.
- Tea tree essential oil applied directly to the site of pain combats infection.

Toothache Poultice

Substitute chaparral in this formula if organically grown goldenseal is not available.

- 2 parts spilanthes powder
- 1 part goldenseal powder (organically cultivated)
- 1 part myrrh powder
- 1 drop clove essential oil

Combine the herb powders with enough water to make a thick paste. Add the clove essential oil as an analgesic and antiseptic. Make a small cylinder-shaped poultice using sterile gauze, and apply directly to the affected area.

Healing Mouthwash

This mouthwash has helped lessen my trips to the dentist. Use daily.

- ¾ cup water
- ¼ cup vodka
- 4 dropperfuls (1 teaspoon) spilanthes tincture
- 2 dropperfuls (½ teaspoon) calendula tincture
- 2 dropperfuls (½ teaspoon) goldenseal (organically culti-vated) or chaparral tincture (see pages 21–23)
- 1 dropperful (¼ teaspoon) myrrh tincture
- 1–2 drops peppermint essential oil

Mix the water and vodka. Add the tinctures and peppermint essential oil and shake well. To use, dilute several tablespoons of the mixture in ½ ounce of water, and use as a mouthwash.

SPLINTERS

WHEN YOU HAVE A SPLINTER, you want to get it out as quickly as you can. Left embedded in the skin, splinters can cause an infection. You can usually unlodge a splinter using a sterilized needle and tweezers. When you have it out, disinfect the area with Kloss's Liniment (see page 93), tea tree essential oil, or a similar disinfectant. If the splinter doesn't come out, you have a few options.

What to Do

You can use any of several techniques to draw the splinter to the surface of the skin, where you can pluck it out. To begin, soak the area in the hottest water you can bear. Adding Epsom salts is helpful, as the salts have a drawing action. Do this several times a day.

If a hot soak doesn't work, apply a thick clay pack (use green or red clay) directly on the spot once or twice a day for several hours.

If a splinter resists to coming out, and the area begins to redden and to feel hot or painful, an infection is taking root. Seek help from a health care professional.

URINARY TRACT INFECTIONS AND CYSTITIS

Cystitis is an infection of the bladder and urinary system. Symptoms include difficult, burning urination; a chronic urge but an inability to urinate; low energy; and sometimes fever. This type of infection can be dangerous if it involves the kidneys, so be mindful and treat it right away.

What to Do

Cystitis and urinary tract infections (UTIs) are generally easy to treat with home remedies. Begin treatment at the first symptoms: a slight burning when urinating, or incomplete emptying of the bladder. If you follow even some of these suggestions, the infection should clear up in a day or two. If it persists for longer than 7 days, consult a holistic health care practitioner.

Rest. Your body is trying to fight off an infection, so slow down and get some rest.

Herbal support. Take herbs used specifically to treat cystitis and UTIs, such as uva ursi, pipsissewa, buchu, cleavers, chickweed, nettle, and dandelion leaf. Combine two or more of these to make a tea; drink several cups a day. Take several teaspoons of echinacea tincture (see pages 21–23) daily to boost your resistance to infection.

Cranberries. Cranberry juice prevents bacteria from adhering to the kidneys and urethra and is one of the best preventives and remedies for urinary tract infections. Drink several cups a day. Unsweetened cranberry juice is best.

Drink water. You need adequate amounts of water when you're suffering from cystitis or a UTI. Fill a quart bottle with water, and add the juice of one or two lemons and a squirt of uva ursi tincture.

Keep the kidney area warm. Don't expose the kidney area to cold water or cold air. Wear long sweaters that cover the kidney area. Place a hot water bottle over your kidneys at night and whenever you're sitting. If you must go to work, take your hot water bottle with you.

Eat a supportive diet. Try lots of yogurt and miso or chicken soup. Alcohol and sugary foods will agitate cystitis, so avoid them. Drink warm teas to soothe the pain and boost the body's natural defenses.

Do not make love. Urinary tract infections are not contagious, but lovemaking can irritate the condition.

Cystitis Remedy

This is an excellent infection-fighting formula for cystitis.

> 2 parts cleavers
> 2 parts fresh or dried cranberries
> 2 parts uva ursi
> 1 part buchu (optional; use if the infection is severe)
> 1 part chickweed
> 1 part marsh mallow root

Mix the herbs and prepare as an infusion, following the instructions on page 12. Drink 4 cups daily, ¼ cup at a time.

WARTS

Warts are viral infections that appear as hard, knotty little protrusions on the skin. Although they are unsightly and annoying, they rarely cause serious problems.

What to Do

Warts are among the most mysterious of all things to treat. They can respond to a plethora of different approaches — from throwing a beefsteak over your left shoulder to burning them off with chemicals. Sometimes they respond to nothing at all. Over the years I've heard a variety of different treatments that have worked for people. Here's a list of some of the most effective treatments:

- The inside of a ripe banana peel applied topically is one recommendation. Tape the inner peel of the banana over the wart; change several times daily. You may have to keep up this treatment for 2 to 3 weeks.
- A poultice of raw eggplant applied topically has been reported to produce excellent results. Change once a day. Again, it may take 2 to 3 weeks.
- Antiviral essential oils such as tea tree, cajeput, and thuja have been applied topically for several weeks with some success.
- A tincture made with equal parts black walnut, echinacea, and pau d'arco is effective if warts are of the spreading type; take ½ teaspoon three times a day, and apply topically as well.
- Kloss's Liniment (see page 93) and cayenne packs placed directly on warts have been successful for me.

RESOURCES

HERB STORES

Herb stores are springing up around the country, and many natural food stores now offer a large selection of herbs. Whenever possible, buy locally. If, however, you are unable to get good-quality herbs close to home, the following sources offer excellent-quality herbs and/or herbal products. Most of these are small mail-order companies owned by herbalists.

Avena Botanicals
207-594-0694
www.avenabotanicals.com

Healing Spirits Herb Farm and Education Center
607-566-2701
www.healingspiritsherbfarm.com

Herb Pharm LLC
800-348-4372
www.herb-pharm.com

Herbalist & Alchemist
908-689-9020
www.herbalist-alchemist.com

Jean's Greens Herbal Tea Works & Herbal Essentials
518-479-0471
www.jeansgreens.com

Mountain Rose Herbs
800-879-3337
www.mountainroseherbs.com

Pacific Botanicals
541-479-7777
www.pacificbotanicals.com

Woodland Essence
315-845-1515
www.woodlandessence.com

Zack Woods Herb Farm
802-851-7536
www.zackwoodsherbs.com

EDUCATIONAL ORGANIZATIONS

American Herb Association
http://ahaherb.com

American Herbalists Guild
617-520-4372
www.americanherbalistsguild.com

California School of Herbal Studies
707-887-7457
www.cshs.com

Herb Research Foundation
www.herbs.org/herbnews

**Sage Mountain Retreat Center &
  Botanical Sanctuary**
802-479-9825
www.sagemountain.com

Tree Farm Communications
800-468-0464
https://treefarmtapes.com

United Plant Savers
740-742-3455
www.unitedplantsavers.org
A nonprofit organization dedicated to the conservation and cultivation of endangered North American medicinal plants. Provides conferences, journals, and other educational services to members.

Metric Conversion Chart

Use the following formulas for converting U.S. measurements to metric. Since the conversions are not exact, it's important to convert the measurements for all of the ingredients to maintain the same proportions as the original recipe.

WHEN THE MEASUREMENT GIVEN IS	MULTIPLY IT BY	TO CONVERT TO
teaspoons	4.93	milliliters
tablespoons	14.79	milliliters
cups	236.59	milliliters
pints	473.18	milliliters
quarts	946.36	milliliters
quarts	0.946	liters
ounces	28.35	grams
inches	2.54	centimeters

INDEX

Page numbers in *italic* indicate illustrations.